201 Tips for Gas or Acidity

& Ulcer, Constipation, Indigestion, Diarrhoea

Dr. Bimal Chhajer
MBBS, MD

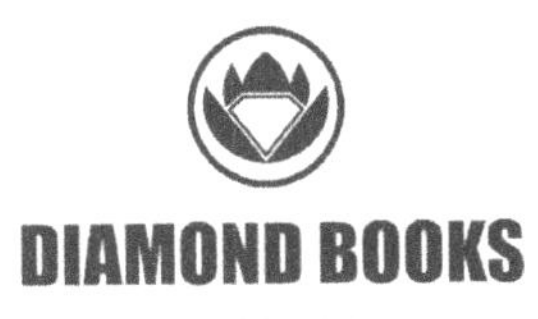

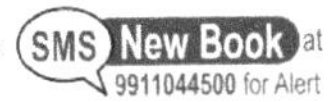

ISBN : 978-93-5083-309-4

Publisher : Diamond Pocket Books (P) Ltd.
X-30, Okhla Industrial Area, Phase-II
New Delhi-110020
Phone : 011-40712200
E-mail : sales@dpb.in
Website : www.diamondbook.in

---

201 Tips for Gas or Acidity

By - *Dr. Bimal Chhajer, MBBS, MD*

Preface

Though I treat heart patients exclusively – I take human body as a whole. So, when I have a heart patient who has a thyroid problem – I try to manage his thyroid as far as possible. When a patient comes with Diabetes – I just do not refer him to a diabetologist but try to control his blood sugar. Heart patients may have problems like sleeplessness, back pain, spondylosis, wehight loss, weight gain, prostate, allergy, nerve pain, knee pain, chest infection – I feel as a allopathy doctor I should put my efforts to solve his associated problems.

One set of very common associated problem for which my patients complain to me is related to the stomach and intestine. This can be Gas, belching, flatus, fowl smelling flatus, bloated abdomen, indigestion, pain in the abdomen, vomiting, loss of appetite, and constipation. Some of the patients have diarrhoea, diarrhoea alternating with constipation; some complain of repeated visits to pass the stool throughout the morning. Out of these thirteen complaints – most come with multiple complaints, some of them have almost all of them. As I have been treating heart patients across the country – south, east, west and north, I have come across these problems more in the eastern part of India.

The general complaints are:

1. **Gas or wind formation**
2. **Belching, acid regurgitation**

3. **Flatus**
4. **Fowl smelling flatus**
5. **Bloated abdomen**
6. **Indigestion**
7. **Pain in abdomen**
8. **Vomiting or nausea**
9. **Loss of appetitie**
10. **Constipation**
11. **Diarrhoea**
12. **Diarrhoea alternating with constipation**
13. **Inability to empty the stool despite repeated visits to the toilet**

All these are related to our Gastro Intestinal System – which includes mainly Oesophagus, Stomach, Intestine (small and large intestine), Liver and Pancreas. Medically if you talk to a doctor or even a gastro intestinal expert – the cause of these symptoms are vague and not clear. Most of the doctors do not take them seriously, some blindly prescribe antacids, give a course of Gastro intestinal antibiotics and try to symptomatically give relief to the patient. If you visit the gastroenterologist (doctors specializing in stomach and intestine) – they would advocate endoscopy and colonoscopy.

If a knowledgeable patient asks the doctors about the medical causes of all these – he or she will say it may be acidity, peptic ulcer, dyspepsia, intestinal fermentation, reflux, indigestion, liver problem, colitis and so on. If a doctor discusses on the causes with another doctor – the diagnosis can be anything ranging from Gastritis, Gastro Esophagial Reflux Disease, gastric ulcer, duodenal ulcer, peptic ulcer, hyper acidity, aerophagy, amoebic or bacterial colitis, hyper or hypomotility of the intestine, irritable bowel syndrome, shortage of enzymes or even chronic dehydration. Sometimes uncommon but serious diseases like Ulcerative colitis, Crohn's disease, intestinal obstruction, malignancy in any part of Gastro Intestinal Tract can also cause the symptoms written above. One very common cause is also side effects of medicines taken for other diseases.

For years I have also treated these complaints/diseases with the medicals drugs, give tit bit tips to my patients on these. But I was inquisitive about why these Gas/wind/flatus/acidity is so common in Kolkata and West Bengal, or for that matter even in Bihar and Bangladesh. No book has given me answer. I discussed with the Naturopathy experts, as they say all the diseases are related to intestine. But no one had any clear cut answer – all vague. This was basically because the medical science has also vague answers to these complaints.

So, when Mr. Narender Verma, my publisher called me for a book on Gas or Acidity I agreed. I would like to recognise the contributions of our dietician Ms. Riburomsuk Nongkynrih and Dr. Roheed Amin, my long term doctor associate in SAAOL for this book.

This book has a lot of names of the drugs to treat the diseases described. But these drugs should not be used by the patients on their own – as a part of self medication. They must consult appropriate medical doctor and get them properly prescribed before they actually use them.

This book has some general knowledge about the Gastro Intestinal System to begin with. Then I have written the common questions on different topics. Every question has been answered keeping in mind that the reader is not a doctor. But being a doctor myself – it is very difficult to avoid using medical terms and phrases. If you find some parts too medical, it is because of my fault in converting medical language to simple language.

–Dr. Bimal Chhajer

MBBS, MD

Contents

Chapter - 1

General Knowledge about the Digestive System

What is Gastro Intestinal Tract?

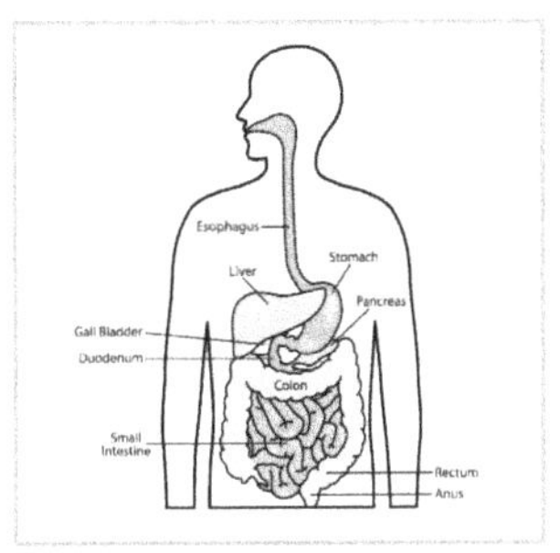

The Gastro Intestinal tract is among the most important organs of the body. The 30+ foot long tube that goes from the mouth to the anus is responsible for the many different body functions. The GI tract is imperative for our wellbeing and our life-long health. The gastrointestinal system is the portal through which nutritive substances, vitamins, minerals, and fluid enter the body. A non-functioning or poorly functioning GI tract can be the source of many chronic health problems that can interfere with your quality of life. In many instances, the death of a person begins in the intestines.

The Gastrointestinal System is responsible for the breakdown and absorption of various foods and liquids needed to sustain life. Many different organs have essential roles in the digestion of food, from the mechanical disrupting by the teeth to the creation of bile (an emulsifier) by the liver. Bile production of the liver plays an important role in digestion: from being stored and concentrated in the gallbladder during fasting stages to being discharged to the small intestine.

What is the GIT composed of?

The gastro intestinal tract includes the mouth, the esophagus, the stomach, the small intestines and large intestine, the rectum and the anus. There are some other organs also that support this digestive process, but are not technically considered part of the digestive system. These organs are the tongue, the glands in the mouth that produce saliva, the pancreas, liver and gallbladder.

What are the functions of the GIT?

The gastro intestinal system performs the following four important functions. It helps to:

1. Store food
2. Mix the food with enzymes produced in different parts of the gastrointestinal tract to break the complex foods to simpler forms of food (digestion).
3. Propel the food mixture through mouth, esophagus, stomach, duodenum, small and large intestines to the anus, and
4. Absorb the various nutrients into the blood especially from small intestine and outer parts.

What does the term digestion mean?

Digestion is the process of breaking down of food into substances that can be absorbed and used by the body for energy, growth and repair.

During digestion, two main processes occur at the same time they are:

Mechanical Digestion: larger pieces of food get broken down into smaller pieces while being prepared for chemical digestion. Mechanical digestion starts in the mouth and continues into the stomach.

Chemical Digestion: starts in the mouth and continues into the intestines. Several different enzymes break down macromolecules into smaller molecules that can be absorbed.

Digestion Process

Mouth

Food is chewed & swallowed saliva contains an enzyme that breaks down starch into glucose.

↓

Esophagus

Food passes down the esophagus to the stomach.

↓

Stomach

The muscle walls of the stomach produce gastric juice that contains protease enzyme. This breaks down protein to amino acids.

↓

Small intestine

Small intestine produces amylase, protease & lipase enzymes to break down additional protein, carbohydrates & fats.

↓

Large intestine

Indigestible food goes to the large intestine.

Water is absorbed and the remaining food becomes faeces.

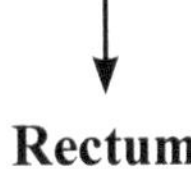

Rectum

Faeces are stored in the rectum and leave the body through the anus.

Where does digestion occur?

As in our body, every part has different and specific function; therefore digestion occurs in the gastrointestinal / digestive tract the 20 to 30 foot long tube extending from your mouth to your anus. Whatever you eat flows through this system, but until it is absorbed through the digestive tract, the nutrients in food are physically outside of your body. Part of the digestion process, then, is the selective transport of nutrients through the cell wall that lines your intestinal tract. Once transported across the intestinal barrier to the inside of your body, these nutrients can enter your bloodstream and circulate to all of your tissues to maintain organ function, support your need for energy, and provide for growth and repair of new cells and tissues.

How does digestion take place in the mouth?

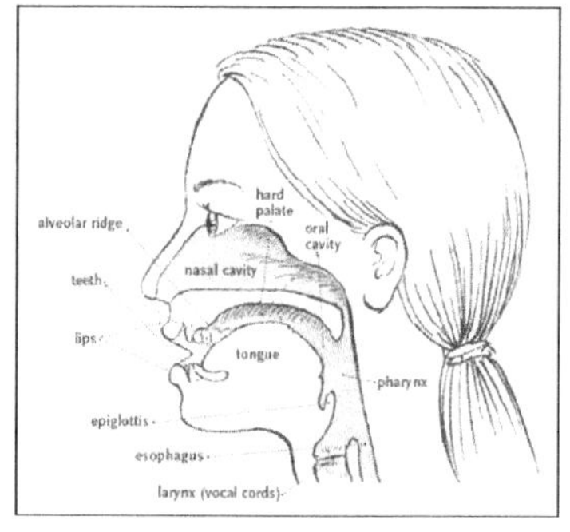

Digestion begins in the mouth with the chewing of food (mastication). That not only breaks down very large groups of food molecules into smaller particles and allows saliva and enzymes to enter inside the larger food complexes, but also sets off a signaling message to the body to start the entire digestive process. After the activation of taste receptors in your mouth and the physical process of mastication, signals the nervous system. For example, the taste of food can trigger the stomach lining to produce acid, therefore, your stomach begins to respond to food even before any food leaves your mouth.

Saliva is secreted by the salivary glands in your mouth and moistens the food to improve the chewing and grinding by teeth. Saliva also contains some enzymes that begin the breakdown of starches and fats to some extent in mouth. For example, carbohydrate digestion begins with the salivary enzyme alpha-amylase, and fat digestion begins with the secretion of the enzyme lingual lipase by glands under your tongue.

Where does saliva come from?

Digestion begins when food enters the mouth and mixes with saliva. A fluid that is 99% water, saliva contains a digestive enzyme called amylase, which breaks down starch foods. The sight, smell, or even the thought of food can trigger the glands to release saliva.

Saliva flows into the mouth from three pairs of large salivary glands: the parotid glands, located just below the ear, the sub maxillary glands in the lower jaw, and the sublingual glands under the tongue. Many smaller salivary glands are also located within the lips, cheeks and tongue. The parotid glands largest of the three secrete saliva into the mouth through tiny openings near the second molar on each side of the upper jaw. The sub maxillary and sub lingual also produces a mucous fluid that helps to make food slippery.

What is the work of an Esophagus?

The esophagus connects the mouth to the stomach. It delivers the saliva-mixed food from the mouth to the stomach and serves as an air lock between the outside world and the digestive tract.

What is bile?

Bile is a thick, bitter, yellow or greenish fluid made in the liver and stored in the gall bladder. Released from the gall blader into the small intestine in response to the presence of food, it is essential to the digestion of fats. It is also a part of the body's excretory or waste disposal system, because it contains the remnants of worn out blood cells. Everyday the liver produces about a litre of bile. It contains a wide range of chemicals including bile salts, mineral salts, cholesterol and bile pigments which gives the bile its own characteristics and colour.

What is a chyme?

After the food has become mixed with the stomach secretions, the resulting mixture that passes down the gut is called chyme. The degree of fluidity of the chyme leaving the stomach depends on the relative amount of food and stomach secretions and on the degree of digestion that has occurred. The appearance of the chyme is that of murky, milky semifluid or paste.

What is the role of the stomach during the process of digestion?

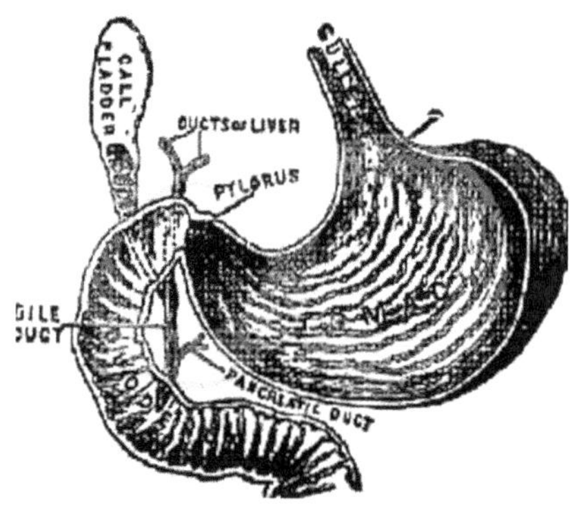

The esophagus opens into the stomach, which is a large chamber. The entire involvement of the stomach in digestion is called the gastric phase of digestion. The stomach is the primary place where proteins are broken down into small parts now known as peptides. Due to its acidic environment, the stomach is also a decontamination chamber that destroys bacteria and other potentially toxic microorganisms that may have entered your digestive system through your mouth.

When the food enters the stomach, the lining of the stomach produces hydrochloric acid (HCl). This acidic environment is critical for destroying toxins in foods, such as bacteria, as well as for untwisting the complex three-dimensional protein chains, a process called denaturation of the proteins.

The stomach lining also secretes the enzyme pepsinogen, which is present in the stomach much of the time but is inactive until the acid (HCl) is present, when it becomes activated as pepsin. Pepsin acts on the denatured proteins by hydrolyzing, or cutting, the bonds between amino acids in the protein chain, resulting in several smaller chains, or peptides.

Fat hydrolysis is very active in the stomach. The fats have already been exposed to lipase in the saliva, which begins the hydrolysis, but it is the gastric lipase, secreted by the stomach, that is primarily responsible for fat hydrolysis in humans.

The antrum, or lower part of the stomach, is the site for the stomach's grinding action and contains a sensor mechanism, called gastrin, for regulating the level of acid produced in the body of the stomach. The antrum also controls the emptying of food into the intestine through the pyloric sphincter. This way the food can be delivered into the intestine in a controlled manner. Once the food-acid-enzyme mixture leaves the stomach, it is called chyme. The movement of chyme through the pyloric sphincter stimulates the intestine to release the hormones secretin and cholecystokinin, which signal the pancreas to release its contents, the pancreatic juice, inside the lumen (the lining) of the duodenum (the first segment of the small intestine).

What does the small intestine comprise of?

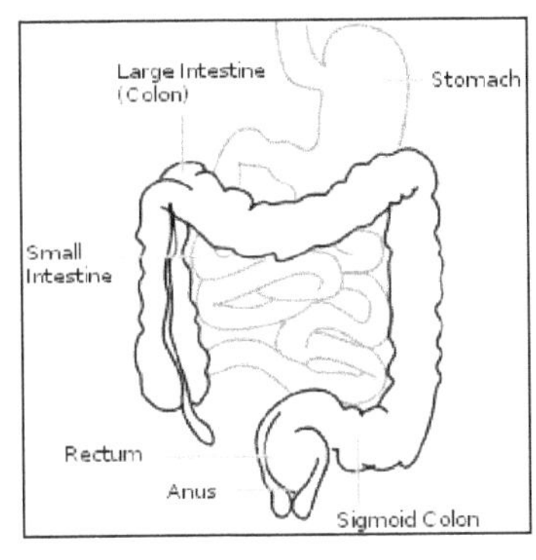

The small intestine is comprise of the duodenum, the part that is closest to the stomach, which helps in neutralization of the bile, the jejunum which is the middle section of the small intestine where most nutrients are actively absorbed and the ileum which is the final part of the small intestine. It is responsible for completing the digestion of nutrients and for reabsorbing the bile salts that have helped to solubilize (keep in solution), the fats.

What is the work of the small intestine?

> Till two years of age a Child has only 20 milk teeth – five in each quadrants. Out of five, one incisor appears at the age of 6 months, the next incisor occurs at the age of 9 months, the canine comes at 18 months, the first and second molars appear at 12 months and 24 months only.

The small intestine, which is specifically designed to maximize the digestion and absorption process, has an expanded surface area with inner folds, called plicae, villi and microvilli, to increase its surface area and enhance its ability to absorb nutrients. All together, this surface is called the brush border of the small intestine. Some enzymes are present on the surface of the brush border, such as disaccharidases like sucrase, maltase, and lactose, which hydrolyze disugars (sugars composed of two monosaccharides) to their two individual sugar molecules.

The duodenum, the part of the small intestine that is closest to the stomach, is a neutralization chamber in which the chyme from the stomach is mixed with bicarbonate, which appears again, this time in the pancreatic juice. Bicarbonate lessens the chyme's acidity, thus allowing more enzymes to function and furthering the breakdown of macromolecules still present. The pancreatic juice also contains many of the enzymes necessary for digestion of proteins, such as trypsin and chymotrypsin, enzymes that cut proteins and peptides down into one-, two-, and three-amino acid chains; and amylase, an enzyme that continues the hydrolysis of starch.

A few nutrients, like iron and calcium, are taken up most efficiently in the duodenum; however, the jejunum, the middle section of the small intestine, is the place where most nutrients are actively absorbed. The amino acids as well as most vitamins and minerals are absorbed in the jejunum. The process of absorption used by the jejunum is called active absorption since your body uses energy to select the exact nutrients it needs. Protein carriers or channels hook-up to these nutrients and take them through the cell wall of the jejunum and into the portal vein, which carries them to the liver.

Active fat absorption also occurs in the duodenum and the jejunum, and requires that the fat to be put into small aggregates that can be transported into your body directly. The body uses bile as a detergent to solubilize the fat. Bile is produced by the liver, stored in the gall bladder, and released into the duodenum and jejunum after a meal. It then can form micelles, small fat droplets, for fat absorption. This process is particularly important for the absorption of the fat-soluble vitamins (vitamins A, D, E, and K), and for cholesterol absorption.

The majority of starch is also digested in the duodenum and jejunum, the first and second segments of the small intestine. The monosaccharide products of carbohydrate digestion, glucose and galactose, are actively absorbed through the intestine by a process that requires energy. Fructose, another common monosaccharide product of carbohydrate digestion, and also a common sweetener for many processed foods, is absorbed more slowly by a process called facilitated transport. Facilitated transport does not require energy.

> The total number of permanent teeth is 32 – eight in each quadrant. Two Incisors(appears at age of 7 and 8); one canine (appears at the age of 11); two pre-molars (appear at the age of 9 and 10) and three molars (appears at the age of 6, 12 and 18 years). Only after 18 that we have 32 teeth.

The ileum is the final part of the small intestine. The ileum is responsible for completing the digestion of nutrients and for reabsorbing the bile salts that have helped to solubilize (keep in solution), the fats. Although most nutrients are absorbed in the duodenum and jejunum, the first two segments of the small intestine, the ileum is the place where vitamin B12 is selectively absorbed into your body.

At the end of transport through the small intestine, the chyme has been depleted of around 90 percent of its vitamins and minerals and the majority of its other nutrients. In addition, around eight to ten liters of fluid is also absorbed in the small intestine each day. Complex carbohydrates that resist the enzyme degradation, such as fiber and resistant starch, remain, as do a small amount of other food molecules and nutrients that have escaped the digestion process. For example, about 3-5% of ingested protein normally escapes digestion and continues to the large intestine.

What happens to the food digested in the large intestine?

The large intestine is not designed for enhancing absorption but is particularly specialized to conserve the sodium and water that escape absorption in the small intestine, although it only transports about one liter of fluid per day. The large intestine is about five feet long, including its final segments, the colon and the rectum.

> Each day, we all usually secrete about 1500 ml of saliva - a watery secretion consisting of mucus and fluid. It contains the enzyme ptyalin that aids digestion and a chemical called lysozyme that acts as a disinfectant to protect the mouth from infection. Saliva is slightly antiseptic.

It is interesting, given that most digestion and absorption occurs prior to the large intestine, that food, which at this point is primarily fiber, will spend more time in your large intestine than anywhere else during digestion. On average, food travels through the stomach in 1/2 to two hours, continues through the small intestine over the next two to six hours, and spends six to 72 hours in your large intestine before final removal by defecation.

One reason food stays longer in the large intestine may be that the large intestine is capable of generating nutrients from food. The food that makes it into the large intestine is primarily fiber, and the large intestine contains an ecosystem of bacteria that can ferment much of this fiber, producing many nutrients necessary for the health of the colon cells. Colonic fermentation also produces a series of short-chain fatty acids, including propionate, acetate, and butyrate, which are required for healthy colonic cell growth and have many other health promoting functions in your body.

How pancreas helps in controlling blood sugar?

The pH of the saliva is 7.0. Its function is to facilitate swallowing, moisten the mouth, serves as a solvent for the molecules that stimulate the taste buds, aids speech by facilitating movements of the lips and tongue and keeps the mouth and teeth clean.

A group of lobe called acini produces four digestive enzymes, these travels through a series of small ducts to the main pancreatic duct. That duct carries the enzymes into the duodenum. Between the acini are group of ductless cells known as Islets of Langerhans, these cells send hormones directly into the blood to control the level of glucose in the body.

The Islets also produce a hormone called glucagons which has the effect of raising rather than lowering the level of sugar in the blood. The purpose of the insulin is to keep the level of sugar in the blood down to normal levels. A lack of this hormone causes diabetes a condition which can be treated with injection of insulin or by diet control. If the level of sugar in the blood begins to rise above certain limits, the Islets of Langerhans respond by releasing insulin into the blood stream. The insulin then acts to oppose the effects of hormones such as cortisone and adrenalin - which raise the level of sugar in the blood.

The insulin exerts its effect by allowing sugar to pass from the bloodstream into the body cells to be used as fuel. But if insulin is absent from the system the mechanism for balancing the blood sugar level is removed, because the sugar in the blood cannot be converted into fuel for the cells then diabetic results.

What does the pancreas do?

The pancreas- tucked neatly into the curve of the duodenum, the first part of the small intestine- behaves like two organs: one releases digestive enzymes to the duodenum and the other releases important hormones to the blood. Because of this dual role- the pancreas is known as both in the exocrine glands and endocrine glands. A group of lobe called acini produces four digestive enzymes, these travels through a series of small ducts to the main pancreatic duct. That duct carries the enzymes into the duodenum. Between the acini are group of ductless cells known as Islets of Langerhans, these cells send hormones directly into the blood to control the level of glucose in the body.

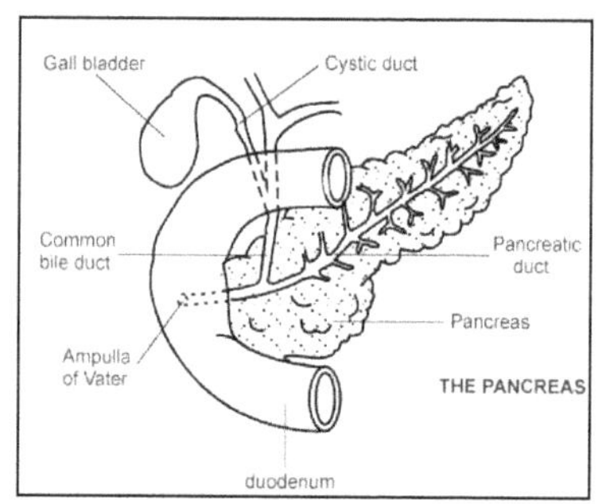

THE PANCREAS

The pancreas also can be thought of as a protein factory. It produces and secretes many of the enzymes necessary for digestion, which include the enzymes that digest protein (trypsin, chymotryosin, carboxypeptidase, and elastase), enzymes that digest fat (lipase and phospholipase), and the enzyme that digests carbohydrate (alpha-amylase). The pancreas releases these enzymes in a pancreatic juice, which is enriched with bicarbonate. The bicarbonate is used to neutralize the acid in chyme. More than a liter of pancreatic juice is released per day in response to signals from eating a meal.

Since your body's tissues are made of protein, the pancreatic enzymes that digest protein have the ability to digest your own tissues. Your body has an intricate protection from self-digestion by these enzymes. The stomach and intestinal tract lining have a mucous layer protecting the tissue from direct digestion by these enzymes. The pancreas uses other mechanisms for protection. Primarily, it produces the enzymes in an inactive form, called zymogens or proenzymes. For example, trypsin is produced as the inactive proenzyme trypsinogen. Trypsinogen is transported to the intestine where it is activated to trypsin by a protease enzyme on the brush border of the intestinal cells. All pancreatic enzymes except lipase and alpha-amylase are secreted as proenzymes, and are therefore inactive within the pancreas.

What are the works of the liver?

The liver is one of the most active organs in your body. The liver is the clearinghouse for all nutrient absorption through the gastrointestinal system. The liver reviews the compounds that have been taken in and has the ability to distinguish toxins and other molecules. It has a detoxification system, in which drugs and toxins are chemically converted to molecules that can be eliminated through the kidneys (urine) or the intestine (stool). The liver is also responsible for synthesizing most of the proteins that circulate in your blood, and it produces bile, which is important for the digestion of fats and is used for the excretion of cholesterol and other fat-soluble molecules.

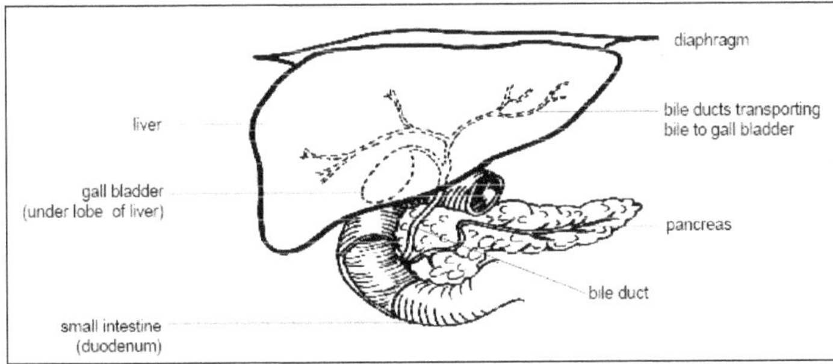

The liver is the major organ involved in maintaining healthy blood sugar (glucose) levels. It monitors your body's glucose needs and provides glucose from digestion, or obtains glucose by breaking down glycogen, the form in which glucose is stored in your liver. The liver has only about a 24-hour supply of glycogen. In prolonged fasting, when glucose is not provided in the diet and glycogen stores have been used, your liver will synthesize glucose from amino acids and other molecules.

The liver is also the primary organ in which fats are metabolized. The liver can make cholesterol and is the primary place where cholesterol is removed from the blood. The liver eliminates cholesterol in the form of bile acids. Every day, your liver secretes about 500 milliliters of bile acids, which are used during digestion to solubilize fats.

How Liver helps in maintaining a health blood sugar?

The liver is the major organ involved in maintaining healthy blood sugar (glucose) levels. It monitors your body's glucose needs and provides glucose from digestion, or obtains glucose by breaking down glycogen, the form in which glucose is stored in your liver. The liver has only about a 24-hour supply of glycogen. In prolonged fasting, when glucose is not provided in the diet and glycogen stores have been used, your liver will synthesize glucose from amino acids and other molecules.

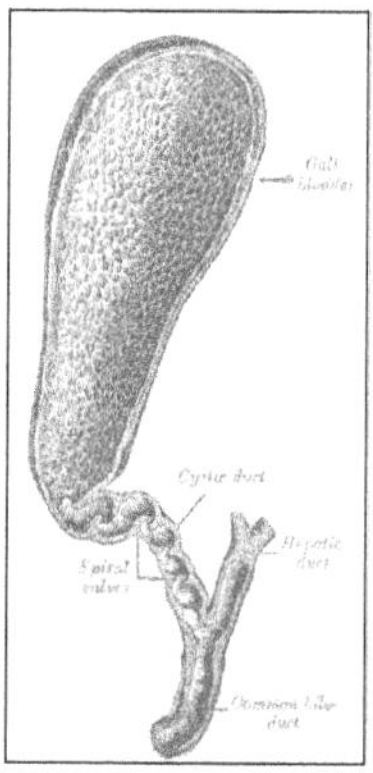

What does the gall bladder do?

The gallbladder is the storage site for the bile acids produced by the liver. After a meal is consumed, the gallbladder is signaled to release its contents into the duodenum and jejunum, where they are available for fat digestion.

What are digestive enzymes and what are the works of the digestive enzyme?

The digestive enzymes are produced by the organs of the digestive tract. They aid in the break down of complex carbohydrates to simple sugars, the fats or lipids to glycerol and fatty acids, and the proteins to amino acids. A distinctive feature of an enzyme is that it is specific those that act on carbohydrates are not capable of acting on fats or protein and vice versa.

What are the different digestive enzymes and where are they present?

Source of the enzyme secretion	Site of enzyme reaction	Name of enzymes and the substances they act upon			
		Starches	Sugar	Fats	Proteins
Salivary glands	Mouth	Salivary amylase (ptyalin)			
Stomach	Stomach			Gastric lipase	Gastric protease (pepsin)
Pancreas	Small intestine	Pancreatic amylase		Pancreatic lipase	Pancreatic proteases
Wall of small intestine	Small intestine		Sucrase Maltase Lactase		Intestinal proteases

How the digestion of carbohydrates takes place in our body?

Carbohydrate digestion which began in the mouth, is resumed in the duodenum. Here nature has provided a second amylase to convert any remaining starch or dextrin to maltose, thus completing the conversion of starch to the disaccharide maltose. Pancreatic amylase appears to be more potent in this action than is salivary amylase. Even uncooked or raw starch, may be digested by pancreatic form of the enzyme. It should be noted that raw starches are less digestible than cooked starches because of the nature of the starch granules. Other carbohydrates, the dissacharides, which are found in the food intake or as end products of amylase action must also be changed to simple sugars before they can be absorbed by the body. The three carbohydrates in the intestinal secretion (sucrose, maltase and lactase) complete the hydrolysis of the carbohydrates to glucose, fructose and galactose.

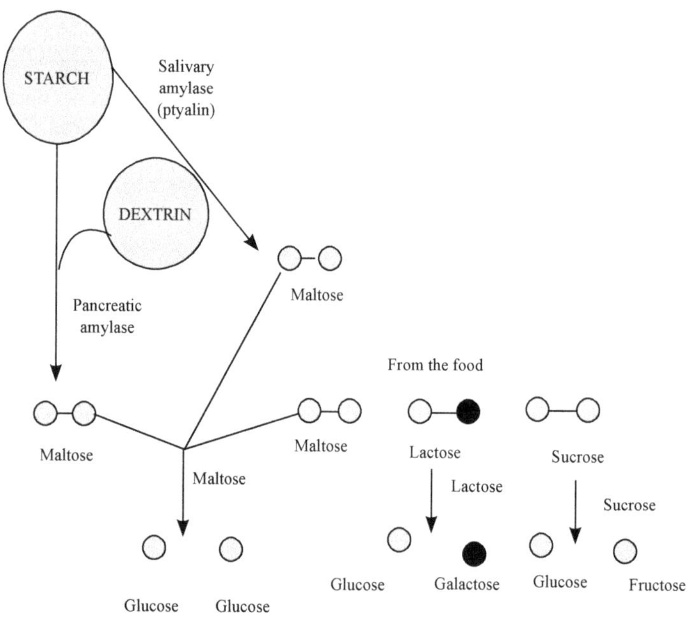

sketch showing Starch & Dissacharide Digestion

How is protein digested in the stomach?

When food enters the stomach it remains temporarily in the upper portion of the organ, though most of the digestive action occurs in the lower part of the stomach. Here the action of the salivary amylase (ptyalin) continues until the pH of the mixture is too acid. Gastric juice, which contains hydrochloric acid, pepsinogen and gastric lipase, is secreted in the lower part of the stomach and is mixed with the food by the churning action of the stomach walls.

Hydrochloric acid plays an important role in gastric digestion. It converts the inactive form of the protein splitting enzyme, pepsinogen to the active enzyme, pepsin; creates the optimum acidity in the stomach for the digestion of protein and acts as a bactericide to prevent the entrance of bacteria into the lower digestive tract. In addition to these functions, hydrochloric acid also may hydrolyze some of the disaccharides contained in the food mass as well as increase the solubility of calcium and iron, which results in the optimum absorption of these essential nutrients in the small intestine.

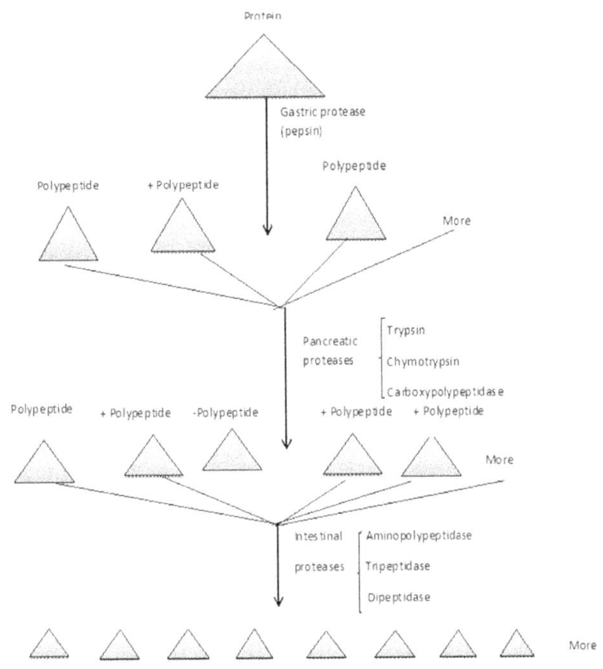

Protein Digestion Sketch

The protein splitting enzyme, pepsin is present in its inactive form, pepsinogen; otherwise when the stomach is empty of food the enzyme would begin to digest the stomach wall. In this first step of protein digestion, the long chain of a protein is split into smaller units called polypeptides by the enzymatic action of pepsin. The polypeptides which vary in size, may contain as few as three amino acids linked together or as many as several hundred. Trypsin is one of the three protein splitting enzymes contributed to the digestive pool by the pancreatic secretion. As in the case of gastric protease (pepsin) trypsin is also secreted in its inactive form, trypsinogen which prevents digestion of the intestinal tissue. Trypsin, chymotrypsin and carboxypolypeptidase attack the links of polypeptide chains and further subdivide them into polypeptides to amino acids is brought about by the action of three additional protein enzymes, aminopeptidase, tripeptidase and dipeptidase, secreted in the intestinal juice.

How is fat digested in the stomach?

A lingual lipase is secreted by Ebner's glands on the dorsal surface of the tongue, and the stomach also secretes a lipase. The gastric lipase is of little importance because there is little enzymatic action produced by gastric lipase, the digestion of fats from the practical standpoint actually begins in the small intestine. The two secretions which are involved in this fat splitting process are the bile, a secretion of the liver, and pancreatic lipase. A fraction of the bile fluid, the bile salts acts as emulsifying agent. The bile also functions to accelerate the action of the pancreatic lipase and to neutralize the acidity of the chyme. In the process of emulsification the fat are broken up into small globules which are easily hydrolysed by pancreatic lipase. Not all of the fat is digested to the glycerol and fatty acid stage by lipase; some of it is hydrolysed only to di-or monoglycerides, which are compounds composed of glycerol and two or one fatty acids repectively.

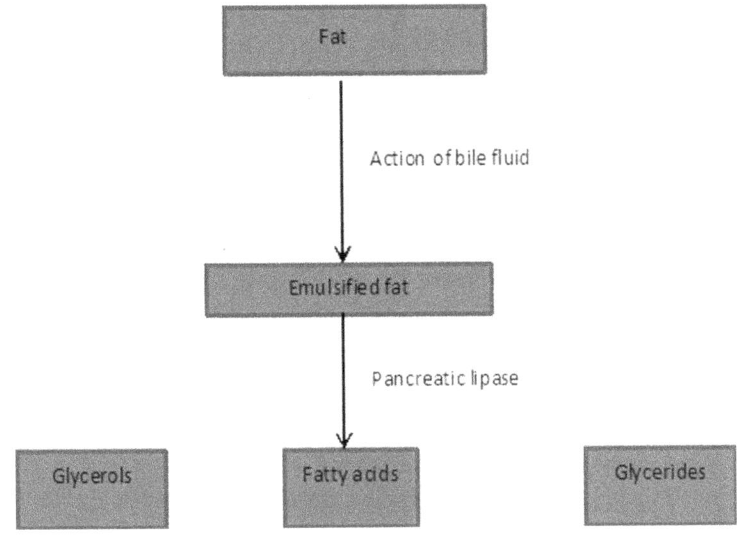

Fat Digestion Sketch

Where are the other nutrients like iron, calcium, vitamins etc absorbed?

A few nutrients, like iron and calcium, are taken up most efficiently in the duodenum; however, the jejunum, the middle section of the small intestine, is the place where most nutrients are actively absorbed. The amino acids as well as most vitamins and minerals are absorbed in the jejunum. The process of absorption used by the jejunum is called active absorption since your body uses energy to select the exact nutrients it needs. Protein carriers or channels hook-up to these nutrients and take them through the cell wall of the jejunum and into the portal vein, which carries them to the liver.

What are the common diseases of Gastrointestinal tract?

Medically speaking the main and common diseases of the gastrointestinal tract can be as follows:

1. Flatulence
2. GERD or Gastro Esophageal Reflux Disease
3. Peptic Ulcer Disease or Acid Peptic Disease
4. Gastritis
5. Dyspepsia or Upper Abdominal Pain or Discomfort
6. Irritable Bowel Syndrome
7. Colitis
8. Constipation and Diarrhoea
9. Diseases of Pancreas and Liver

What are the areas of the abdomen and what diseases they are related to?

Shown in the diagram are the areas of the abdomen, and the most likely underlying pathology.

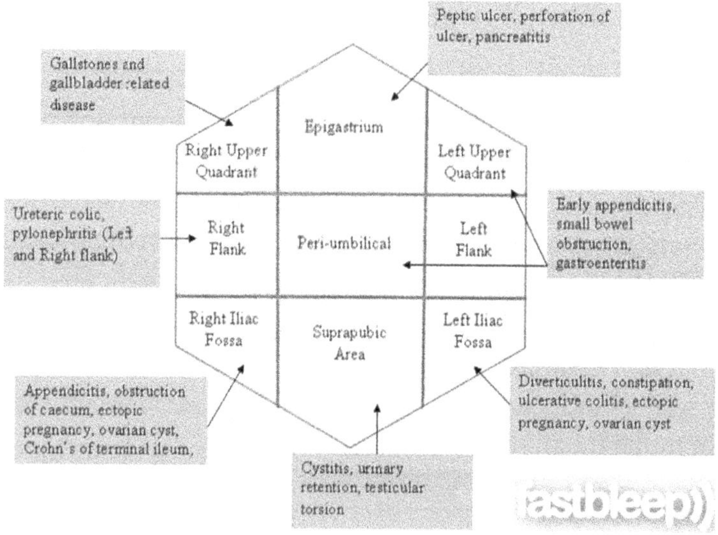

Chapter - 2

Gas & Flatulence

Q 1. What is Flatulence ?

Flatulence is the expulsion through the rectum of a mixture of gases that are by-products of the digestion process of mammals and other animals. The medical term for the mixture of gases is flatus, informally known as a fart, or simply gas. The gases are expelled from the rectum in a process colloquially referred to as "passing gas", "breaking wind" or "farting". Flatus is brought to the rectum by the same peristaltic process which causes feces to descend from the large intestine. The noises commonly associated with flatulence are caused by the vibration of the anal sphincter, and occasionally by the closed buttocks. Many a times this also called "Wind Formation".

Q 2. What is Belching ?

It is the expulsion of the gas or air from the mouth, mostly accompanied with loud sound. This air that comes out are mostly swallowed air present in the stomach. But when associated with Gastritis or Acid Peptic Disease or food intolarence – this gas comes out with a bitter tasting liquid (mostly acid, gastric juice from the stomach). This may also be called Regurgitation or Waterbrash. Many a times this problem is called as "Gas Formation".

Q 3. In Flatulence what is the composition of this gas and where it comes from?

Gas is made primarily of odourless vapours – Carbon dioxide, Oxygen, Nitrogen, Hydrogen and sometimes Methane. The unpleasant odour of flatulence comes from bacteria in the large intestine that release small amounts of gases that contain sulphur.

Most gases in the stomach are mixtures of nitrogen and oxygen derived from swallowed air and most of these gases are expelled by belching.

> Swallowing is initiated by the voluntary action of collecting the oral contents on the tongue and propelling them backward into the pharynx. The total number of swallows per day is about 2400.

Only small amount of gas are normally present in the small intestine and much of this gas is air that passes from the stomach into the intestinal tract. In addition, considerable amount of carbon dioxide occasionally accumulate because reaction between acidic gastric juice and bicarbonate in pancreatic juice sometimes liberates carbon dioxide too rapidly for all of this to be absorbed.

In the large intestine, a greater proportion of the gases is derived from bacterial action, including especially carbon dioxide, methane and hydrogen. They occur along with varying amount of oxygen and nitrogen from swallowed air.

Although having gas is common, it can be uncomfortable and embarrassing. Understanding causes, ways to reduce symptoms and treatment will help most people find relief.

Q 4. Passing Gas or Wind – is it a disease?

A healthy man has 100-200ml of gas in the digestive tract at any time. Passing of about 500 ml of gas per day is very normal.

This may increase to 2-3 litres when the colon bacteria leads to fermentation of the fibre or undigested carbohydrate. This is not a disease and it can be called a food intolarence. An average person can normally pass about 10-14 times flatus per day.

Q 5. What is the reaction of people to flatus socially?

When a small survey was carried on the social implications in USA – 47 % people thought that flatus is a natural event and they were comfortable with it; 21% did not like flatus but thought it was accepted in society; 32% were embarrassed by sound, smell of flatus.

This flatulence is common in as many as 75% population in Asians and Blacks.

Q 6. What is the cause of different types of gases in the intestine or flatus?

The composition of the flatus varies widely depending on the diet and bacterial fermentation. If the flatus is due to swallowed air the composition will be like the inhaled air (20% oxygen, 70-80% Nitrogen).

If the gas is produced by fermentation of the undigested carbohydrate foods is almost exclusively in the small and large intestine – the gas produced is Hydrogen. As this gas can also come out of the mouth in the form of belching – the hydrogen content of the gas can be measured by a test.

Carbon dioxide gas can be produced due to neutralization of the acid by bicarbonate present in the intestinal juices. Bacterial fermentation of fats and proteins can also increase the carbon dioxide content of the flatus. Large amount of germs or bacteria is always present in the large intestine and they ferment the undigested foods passing through the intestine.

Methane gas can be produced by the fermenatation of undigested carbohydrates by a particular bacteria, Methanobrevibactor smithii, which try to break carbohydrates, proteins, glycoproteins without consuming oxygen.

Q 7. Sometimes the flatus is full of fowl smelling gas. What is the cause?

When the foods contain sulphur – they are fermented producing gases like Hydrogen Sulphide, methanethiol, dimethyl sulphide. These three are thought to be most odour producing gases. Ammonia, amines, skatoles and indols may contribute to the odor as well. Very little amount of hydrogen sulphide (three in 10 lac) also can lead to a detectable smell in the flatus. Eating some sulphur containing salts (kala namak), onions and garlic also leads to release of these gases.

Q 8. What are the mechanisms that the gases are produced?

Gas in the digestive tract (that is, the esophagus, stomach, small intestine, and large intestine) comes from two sources:

1. Swallowed air
2. Normal breakdown of certain undigested foods by harmless bacteria naturally present in the large intestine (colon)

Q 9. Do we swallow this air that come out in the flatus or belching?

Air swallowed (aerophagia) is a common cause of gas in the stomach. Everyone swallows small amount of air when eating and drinking. However, eating or drinking rapidly, chewing gum, eating hard candy, smoking cigarettes/bidi, drinking through straws, drinking carbonated drinks like cola/pepsi, dry mouth or wearing loose dentures can cause some people to take in more air. Anxiety and rapid breathing can also lead to swallowing of air.

> The palate is the roof of the mouth which is made up of the parts which separate the mouth from the nasal cavity. It consists of the hard palate and the soft palate.

Burping or belching is the process by which most swallowed air, which contains nitrogen, oxygen and carbon dioxide, leaves the stomach. The remaining gas moves into the small intestine where it is partially absorbed. A small amount travels into the large intestine for release through the rectum. (The stomach also releases carbon dioxide when stomach acid and bicarbonate mix but most of this gas is absorbed into the bloodstream and does not enter the large intestine.)

Q 10. What is the cause of production of the gases in the intestine?

The body does not digest and absorb some carbohydrates (the sugar, starches and fiber found in many foods) in the small intestine because of shortage or absence of certain enzymes.

This undigested food then passes from the small intestine into the large intestine where normal, harmless bacteria break down the food, producing hydrogen, carbon dioxide and in about one-third of all people methane. Eventually these gases exit through the rectum.

Q 11. What are the other symptoms and problems associated with gas?

The most common symptoms of gas are flatulence, abdominal bloating, abdominal pain, and belching. However, not everyone experiences these symptoms. The type and degree of symptoms probably depends on how much gas the body produces, how many fatty acids the body absorbs, and a person's sensitivity to gas in the large intestine.

Q 12. Why belching and flatulence come together?

Flatulence is closely related to belching and bloating. The gas, produced in the upper part of the intestine, often pass upwards – cross the stomach and esophagus and come out from the mouth. This gas often gets stored in the stomach leading to discomfort.

Belching requires the sphingter (door) between the stomach and esophagus to open and this can be controlled by us. Release of air after food often releases fullness and distension of the stomach is known as "Megenblase Syndrome" and gives a relief to many people.

Q 13. What diagnostic tests are used to find the cause of gas?

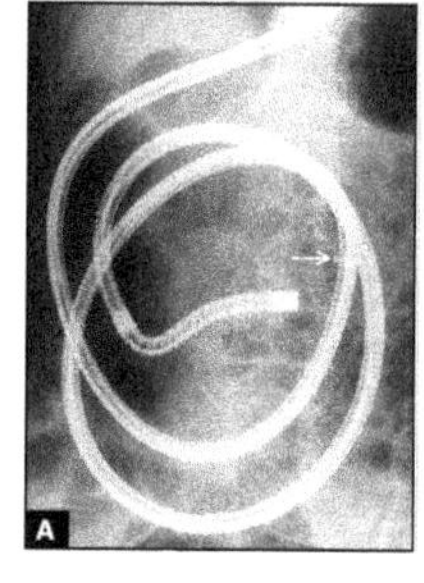

Because gas symptoms may be caused by a serious disorder, those causes should be ruled out. Health professionals usually begin with a review of dietary habits and symptoms. The health professional may ask the patient to keep a diary of foods and beverages consumed for a specific time period. If lactase deficiency is the suspected cause of gas, the health professional may suggest avoiding milk products for a period of time. A blood or breath test may be used to diagnose lactose intolerance. In addition, to determine if someone produces too much gas in the colon or is unusually sensitive to the passage of normal gas volumes, the health professional may ask a patient to count the number of times he passes gas during the day and include this information in a diary. Careful review of diet and the amount of gas passed may help relate specific foods to symptoms and determine the severity of the problem.

Because the symptoms are so variable, the health professional may order other types of diagnostic tests in addition to a physical exam, depending on the patient's symptoms and other factors.

> Pharynx is the first part of the digestive canal after the mouth. It is about 12 cm long. It also has voice box in the front which is connected to the digestive canal by a hole which has a lid. If we talk during swallowing – this lead opens and food particle can go into the voice box. This leads to a severe cough reflex throwing the food back again from the voice box. So, we should not talk while eating.

Q. 14. Which foods cause gas?

Most foods that contain carbohydrates can cause gas. By contrast, fats and proteins cause little gas.

Sugars:

The sugars that cause gas are raffinose, lactose, fructose, and sorbitol.

Raffinose:

Beans contain large amounts of this complex sugar. Smaller amounts are found in cabbage, brussels sprouts, broccoli, asparagus, other vegetables, and whole grains.

Lactose:

Lactose is the natural sugar in milk. It is also found in milk products, such as cheese and ice cream, and processed foods, such as bread, cereal, and salad dressing. Many people, particularly those of African, Native American, or Asian background, normally have low levels of lactase, the enzyme needed to digest lactose, after childhood. Also, as people age, their enzyme levels decrease. As a result, over time people may experience increasing amounts of gas after eating food containing lactose.

Fructose:

Fructose is naturally present in onions, artichokes, pears, and wheat. It is also used as a sweetener in some soft drinks and fruit drinks.

Sorbitol:

Sorbitol is a sugar found naturally in fruits, including apples, pears, peaches, and prunes. It is also used as an artificial sweetener in many dietetic foods and sugar-free candies and gums.

Starches:

Most starches, including potatoes, corn, pasta, and wheat, produce gas as they are broken down in the large intestine. Rice is the only starch that does not cause gas.

Fiber:

Many foods contain soluble and insoluble fiber. Soluble fiber dissolves easily in water and takes on a soft, gel-like texture in the intestines. Found in oat bran, beans, peas, and most fruits, soluble fiber is not broken down until it reaches the large intestine, where digestion causes gas.

Insoluble fiber, on the other hand, passes essentially unchanged through the intestines and produces little gas. Wheat bran and some vegetables contain this kind of fiber.

Q 15. What are the other causes of production of gases in the gut and flatulence?

Apart from swallowing of air, lactose intolerance, undigested food getting fermencted – flatulence can be cause by Irritable bowel syndrome (a very common stress related disease) and drugs. Excessive bacterial growth in the intestine due to colitis is also a major cause of flatulence. Peptic ulcer, infection in the intestine, gall stones, intestinal inflammation, hypo thyroidism, malignancy in the colon can also cause flatulence.

Q 16. What are the drugs that lead to Flatulence?

Many of the allopathic drugs can lead to abdominal distress and gas formation. Antibiotics, anticholinergics (used to treat abdominal pain), antidiarrheals, calcium channel blockers, fibric acid derivatives are some of the common drugs that can lead to gas formation.

Q. 17. Can consumption of milk lead to flatus formation?

Milk contains lactose and an enzyme called lactase helps to break this lactose in the intestine. Many people, especially the adults, do not have this milk digesting enzyme. It is known that the amount of lactase decreases with age – 10% of lactase activity is lost by the age of 20. This leads to lot of intestinal fermentation of milk and production of flatus. This is popularly called Lactose Intolerance. Lactose intolerance is often accompanied by abdominal pain, distension, loose watery stools and cramping.

Q 18. Tell us more about Milk intolerance, since milk is a major content of our food.

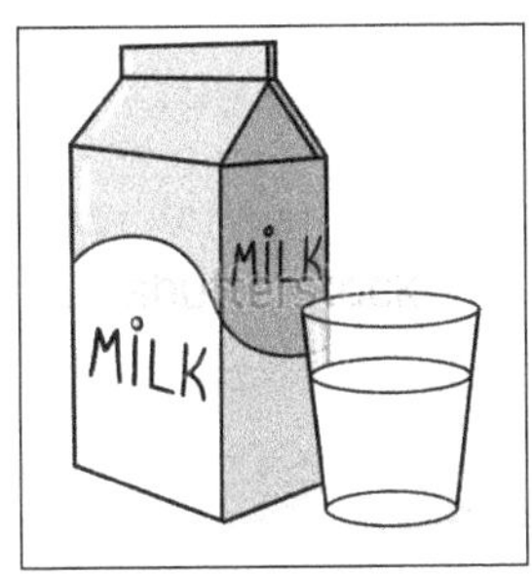

Lactose intolerance is the inability to digest and absorb lactose (the sugar in milk) that results in gastrointestinal symptoms when milk or food products containing milk are consumed. Lactose intolerance happens when the small intestine does not make enough of the enzyme lactase. Enzymes help the body absorb foods. Not having enough lactase is called lactase deficiency. Babies' bodies make this enzyme so they can digest milk, including breast milk. Premature babies sometimes have lactose intolerance. Children who were born at full term usually do not show signs of lactose intolerance until they are at least 3 years old. Lactose intolerance can begin at different times in life. In Caucasians, it usually affects children older than age 5. In African Americans, lactose intolerance often occurs as early as age 2. Lactose intolerance is more common in people with Asian, African, Native American, or Mediterranean ancestry than it is among northern and western Europeans. Lactose intolerance is very common in adults and is not dangerous. Approximately 30 million American adults have some amount of lactose intolerance by age 20.

Epiglottis is a flap of tissue at the entrance to the larynx or airway. When food is being swallowed this flap is pushed across the opening so that the food cannot be pushed down into the lungs, causing choking.

Q. 19. Can milk intolerance develop also in children?

Lactase deficiency may occur because of a congenital absence (absent from birth) of lactase due to a mutation in the gene that is responsible for producing lactase. This is a very rare cause of lactase deficiency, and the symptoms of this type of lactase deficiency begin shortly after birth.

Q.20-21. Why lactose or milk intolerance occurs in adults? How it develops with age?

The most common cause of lactase deficiency is a decrease in the amount of lactase that occurs after childhood and persists into adulthood, referred to as adult-type hypolactasia. This decrease in lactase is genetically programmed, and the prevalence of this type of lactase deficiency in different ethnic groups is highly variable. Thus, in Asian populations it is almost 100%, among American Indians it is 80%, and in Blacks it is 70%; however, in American Caucasians the prevalence of lactase deficiency is only 20%. In addition to variability in the prevalence of lactase deficiency, there also is variability in the age at which symptoms of lactose intolerance appear. Thus, in Asian populations, the symptoms of lactase deficiency (intolerance) occur around the age of 5, among Blacks and Mexican-Americans by the age of 10, and in the Finnish by age 20.

> The esophagus – or the food pipe connects the Pharynx to the stomach. It is 25cm long muscular tube which passes the chest behind the heart and crosses the diaphragm to open in the stomach. The distance of the junction of the esophagus and stomach from the teeth is 40cm. The swallowed food crosses this distance in less than a minute.

It is important to emphasize that lactase deficiency is not the same as lactose intolerance. Persons with milder deficiencies of lactase often have no symptoms after the ingestion of milk. For unclear reasons, even persons with moderate deficiencies of lactase may not have symptoms. A diagnosis of lactase deficiency is made when the amount of lactase in the intestine is reduced, but a diagnosis of lactose intolerance is made only when the reduced amount of lactase causes symptoms.

Q 22. What may be the difficulties when we should suspect Milk Intolerance?

Common symptoms linked to lactose intolerance include:

1. Anorexia and nausea
2. Intestinal distension
3. Abdominal cramps
4. Gas and flatulence
5. Severe diarrhoea
6. Under nutrition and loss of weight

Unfortunately, these symptoms can be caused by several gastrointestinal conditions or diseases, so the presence of these symptoms is not very good at predicting whether a person has lactase deficiency or lactose intolerance.

Symptoms occur because the unabsorbed lactose passes through the small intestine and into the colon. In the colon, one type of normal bacterium contains lactase and is able to split the lactose and use the resulting glucose and galactose for its own purposes. Unfortunately, when they use the glucose and galactose, these bacteria also release hydrogen gas. Some of the gas is absorbed from the colon and into the body and is then expelled by the lungs in the breath. Most of the hydrogen, however, is used up in the colon by other bacteria. A small proportion of the hydrogen gas is expelled and is responsible for the increased flatulence (passing gas). Some people have an additional type of bacterium in their colons that changes the hydrogen gas into methane gas, and these people will excrete only methane or both hydrogen and methane gas in their breath and flatus.

> When in erect position and when it contains a small amount of liquid stomach is a J shaped bag; the vertical stack of the J forms upper two third of the stomach(called the body of the stomach), which is surmounted by a convex cap, called the Fundus, and the lower one third is called the Pyloric part of the stomach.

Not all of the lactose that reaches the colon is split and used by colonic bacteria. The unsplit lactose in the colon draws water into the colon (by osmosis). This leads to loose, diarrheal stools.

The severity of the symptoms of lactose intolerance varies greatly from person to person. One reason for this variability is that people have different amounts of lactose in their diet; the more lactose in the diet, the more likely and severe the symptoms. Another reason for the variability is that people have differing severities of lactase deficiency, that is, they may have mild, moderate, or severe reduction in the amounts of lactase in their intestines. Thus, small amounts of lactose will cause major symptoms in severely lactase deficient people but only mild or no symptoms in mildly lactase deficient people. Finally, people may have different responses to the same amount of lactose reaching the colon. Whereas some may have mild or no symptoms, others may have moderate symptoms. The reason for this is not clear but may relate to differences in their intestinal bacteria.

Q23. How to confirm lactose intolerance with medical tests?

Other intestinal problems, such as irritable bowel syndrome, may cause the same symptoms as lactose intolerance.

Tests to help diagnose lactose intolerance include:

- Enteroscopy
- Lactose-hydrogen breath test
- Lactose tolerance test
- Stool pH

Q 24. Any easier way to diagnose Milk Intolerance?

Elimination diet

Probably the most common way that people self-diagnose lactose intolerance is by an elimination diet, a diet that eliminates milk and milk products. There are several problems with this type of "testing."

1. Milk products are so common in prepared foods from the supermarket or restaurant that it is likely that an elimination diet that is not rigorous (i.e., does not eliminate all milk-containing products) will still include substantial amounts of milk. Thus, persons with severe lactase deficiency attempting an elimination diet may be ingesting enough lactose to have symptoms and erroneously conclude that lactose intolerance is not responsible for the symptoms.

2. People often make the assumption that they are lactose intolerant based on a short trial of elimination. A short trial may be adequate if symptoms are severe and occurring daily, but not if the symptoms are subtle and/or variable. In the latter case, an elimination diet may need to be continued for several weeks.
3. Because symptoms of lactose intolerance are subjective and variable, there is always a possibility of a "placebo effect" in which people think they feel better eliminating milk when, in fact, they are no better. As discussed previously, with subjective symptoms such as those of lactose intolerance, a placebo effect might be expected to occur 20%-40% of the time.

The Duodenum (25cm in length) is a "C" shaped first part of the small intestine which connects the stomach and intestine. Two very important tubes join together and open into this part – the Bile duct and Pancreatic duct. They bring Liver Juice (bile) and Pancreatic Juice to digest the food particles.

If an elimination diet is to be used for diagnosing lactose intolerance, it should be a rigorous diet. A rigorous diet requires counseling by a dietician or reading a guide to a lactose-elimination diet. The diet also needs to be continued long enough to clearly evaluate whether or not symptoms are better. If there is doubt about improvement on the diet, particularly if symptoms normally fluctuate in intensity over weeks or months, repeated periods of lactose elimination should be tried until a firm conclusion can be drawn. Elimination of all milk products should eliminate symptoms completely if lactose intolerance alone is the cause of the symptoms.

Q 25. Can we give milk and see if flatulence occurs?

A milk challenge is a simpler way of diagnosing lactose intolerance than an elimination diet. A person fasts overnight and then drinks a glass of milk in the morning. Nothing further is eaten or drunk for 3-5 hours. If a person is lactose intolerant, the milk should produce symptoms within several hours of ingestion. If there are no symptoms or symptoms are substantially milder than the usual symptoms, it is unlikely that lactose intolerance is the cause of the symptoms. It is important that the milk that is used is fat-free in order to eliminate the possibility that fat in the milk is the cause of symptoms. It is not possible to eliminate the possibility that symptoms are due to milk allergy, a very different condition than lactose intolerance; however, this usually is not confusing since allergy to milk is rare and primarily occurs in infants and young children. (If milk allergy is a consideration, pure lactose can be used instead of milk.)

> After Duodenum(25 cm long), the rest of the small intestine can be up to 23 feet in length – and has two parts – Jejunum (first 40%) and Ileum (last 60%). From here only, the digested food is absorbed into the blood stream.

An important issue is the amount of milk required for the milk challenge.

- If a person drinks several glasses of milk or ingests large amounts of milk-containing products in their normal diet, then a larger amount of milk should be used in the challenge, 8-16 ounces in an adult, equivalent to one or two large glasses of milk.
- If the person being tested usually does not drink several glasses of milk or ingest larger quantities of milk-containing products, there may be a problem with using 8-16 ounces of milk for testing. These larger quantities of milk used for testing may cause symptoms, but the smaller amounts of milk or milk products that these persons ingest in their normal diet may not be enough to cause symptoms. Technically, they may be lactose intolerant when they are tested with larger amounts of milk, but lactose in their normal diet cannot be responsible for their usual symptoms.

Q 26. What are the other sources of lactose in the diet?

Although milk and foods made from milk are the only natural sources of lactose, lactose often is "hidden" in prepared foods to which it has been added. People with very low tolerance for lactose should know about the many food products that may contain lactose, even in small amounts. Food products that may contain lactose include:

- bread and other baked goods;
- processed breakfast cereals;
- instant potatoes, soups, and breakfast drinks;
- margarine;
- lunch meats (except those that are kosher);
- salad dressings;
- candies and other snacks; and
- mixes for pancakes, biscuits, and cookies.

Some products labeled nondairy, such as powdered coffee creamer and whipped toppings, also may include ingredients that are derived from milk and, therefore, contain lactose.

Smart shoppers learn to read food labels with care, looking not only for milk and lactose in the contents but also for such words as whey, curds, milk by-products, dry milk solids, and nonfat dry milk powder. If any of these are listed on a label, the item contains lactose.

In addition to food sources, lactose can be "hidden" in medicines. Lactose is used as the base for more than 20% of prescription drugs and about 6% of over-the-counter drugs. Many types of birth control pills, for example, contain lactose, as do some tablets used for stomach acid and gas. However, these products typically affect only people with severe lactose intolerance because they contain such small amounts of lactose.

Q 27. How is lactose intolerance treated?

Dietary changes:

The jejunum is attached to the back of the abdominal wall by a fan-like structure called the mesentery which is made up of two layers of peritoneum. It is while food is in the jejunum that its nutritive elements are absorbed into the blood. For this reason the jejunum has a highly efficient blood supply carried in numerous arteries and veins.

The most obvious means of treating lactose intolerance is by reducing the amount of lactose in the diet. Fortunately, most people who are lactose intolerant can tolerate small or even moderate amounts of lactose. It often takes only elimination of the major milk-containing products to obtain sufficient relief from their symptoms. Thus, it may be necessary to eliminate only milk, yogurt, cottage cheese, and ice cream. Though yogurt contains large amounts of lactose, it often is well-tolerated by lactose intolerant people. This may be so because the bacteria used to make yogurt contain lactase, and the lactase is able to split some of the lactose during storage of the yogurt as well as after the yogurt is eaten (in the stomach and intestine). Yogurt also has been shown to empty more slowly from the stomach than an equivalent amount of milk. This allows more time for intestinal lactase to split the lactose in yogurt, and, at least theoretically, would result in less lactose reaching the colon.

The ileum is the lower part of the small intestine, and is the part which the food reaches last on its way from the stomach to the colon, or large bowel. It is a 3.5 m (2 ft) long tube-leading on from the duodenum and the jejunum and connecting with the large intestine.

Most supermarkets carry milk that has had the lactose already split by the addition of lactase. Substitutes for milk also are available, including soy and rice milk. Acidophilus-containing milk is not beneficial since it contains as much lactose as regular milk, and acidophilus bacteria do not split lactose.

For individuals who are intolerant to even small amounts of lactose, the dietary restrictions become more severe. Any purchased product containing milk must be avoided. It is especially important to eliminate prepared foods containing milk purchased from the supermarket and dishes from restaurants that have sauces.

> The large intestine is about 1.5 meter (5 feet) and has seven parts starting from front to end. They are Caecum, ascending colon, transverse colon, decending colon, sigmoid colon, rectum and anal canal respectively.

Another means to reduce symptoms of lactose intolerance is to ingest any milk-containing foods during meals. Meals (particularly meals containing fat) reduce the rate at which the stomach empties into the small intestine. This reduces the rate at which lactose enters the small intestine and allows more time for the limited amount of lactase to split the lactose without being overwhelmed by the full load of lactose at once. Studies have shown that the absorption of lactose from whole milk, which contains fat, is greater than from non-fat milk, perhaps for this very reason. Nevertheless, the substitution of whole milk or yogurt for non-fat milk or yogurt does not seem to reduce the symptoms of lactose intolerance.

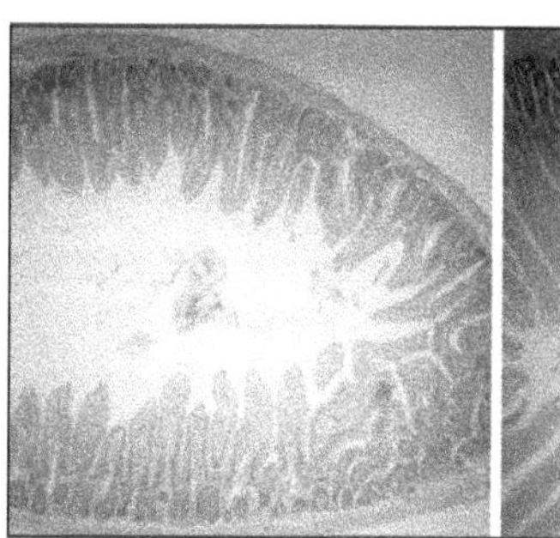
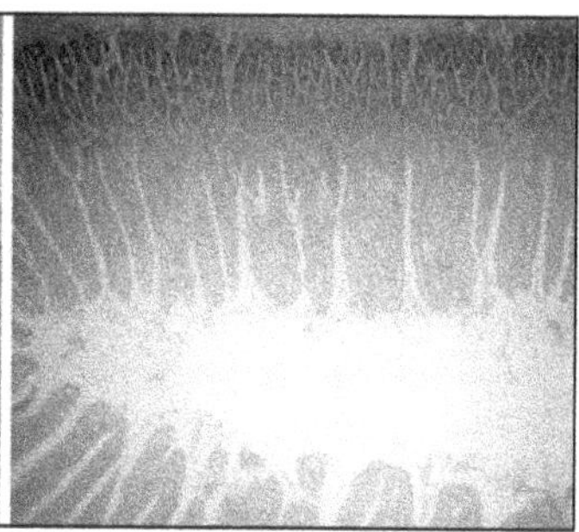

Lactase enzyme:

Caplets or tablets of lactase are available to take with milk-containing foods.

Adaptation:

Some people find that by slowly increasing the amount of milk or milk-containing products in their diets they are able to tolerate larger amounts of lactose without developing symptoms. This adaptation to increasing amounts of milk is not due to increases in lactase in the intestine. Adaptation probably results from alterations in the bacteria in the colon. Increasing amounts of lactose entering the colon change the colonic environment, for example, by increasing the acidity of the colon. These changes may alter the way in which the colonic bacteria handle lactose. For example, the bacteria may produce less gas. There also may be a reduction in the secretion of water and, therefore, less diarrhoea.

Calcium and Vitamin D supplements:

Milk and milk-containing products are the best sources of dietary calcium, so it is no wonder that calcium deficiency is common among lactose intolerant persons. This increases the risk and severity of osteoporosis and the resulting bone fractures. It is important, therefore, for lactose intolerant persons to supplement their diets with calcium. A deficiency of vitamin D also causes disease of the bones and fractures. Milk is fortified with vitamin D and is a major source of vitamin D for many people. Although other sources of vitamin D can substitute for milk, it is a good idea for lactose-intolerant persons to take supplemental vitamin D to prevent vitamin D deficiency.

Q. 28. Why the flatulence problem is increasing?

With more and more people knowing the bad effects of fatty food and good effects of carbohydrates with more fiber – many have started consuming more fruits and vegetables. They do so in order to treat Coronary Heart Disease, Diabetes, High Blood Pressure and Cancer. This indirectly have increased flatulence problem.

Q 29. What are the tests that can be done on patients with excess gas formation, flatulence?

a. A complete blood examination with cell count (TLC, DLC), electrolytes, blood glucose, liver function tests including albumin and protein should be checked first. They are done to diagnose infection, diabetes, malabsorption, cancer, cirrhosis of liver and possible infection.

b. Stool should be checked for undigested foods and parasites. Amebiaisi, Giardiasis can be excluded with such check up. Fat content of the stool can also be checked.

c. X-ray of the abdomen should be done to see how much gas is present. Distension of the colon, obstruction, free air can be diagnosed with this test.

d. Endoscopy or colonoscopy are little invasive tests and should be avoided if the case is not so severe. But in severe cases and chronic cases these investigation can give invaluable leads for diagnosis.

e. Breath tests: Hydrogen breath test can diagnose lactose intolerance very clearly. Carbon Dioxide tests can lead to diagnosis of excess fermentation in the gut.

Q30. How to treat flatulence?

Treatment of Flatulence or gas problem falls in three categories:

a. Treatment of aerophagy or swallowing of air

b. Treatment by diet behaviour modification

c. Treatment with medicines

d. Treatment by Naturopathy and Yoga

Q 31. How to treat air swallowing?

If the person has a lot of belching due to swallowed air – asking them the tips to eat will improve the belching or passage of gas through the mouth. These are eating and drinking slowly, not to eat while lying down, avoiding chewing gum and hard candies, avoid drinking liquids with straws, avoid carbonated drinks and coffee.

Q. 32. What should be the diet behaviour modification treatment for gas or flatulence?

Diet behaviour modification would be to find out which kind of foods are leading to more flatulence and try avoid them.

a. They should try to eliminate and reintroduce the following foods and see if they are related to increased flatulence. If introducing them increases flatulence and exclusion decreases flatulence – the culprit food should be eliminated from the food. This can also be called Elimination diet.

1. Milk and milk products
2. Fruits: Apple, Banana, figs, pears, melons, oranges, raisins and other fruits
3. Vegetables: all leafy vegetable, cabbage, carrots, broccoli, cauliflower, beans, garlic, onion
4. Cereals: Bran, oat, corn, soya beans
5. Others: Fructose containing foods, nuts (ground nuts, coconut, Cachew nuts), Fish, chicken, red meat, popcorn, avocado, rice, wheat with Gluten, eggs, non milk Chocolates.

b. Many salads when taken can cause Flatus formation – boiled salads/ *subjees* can be taken with much reduction of flatus.

c. Sprouted beans and pulses also cause Flatus and belching in many – they can be taken after steaming or boiling.

d. Removal of all fibers in the diet can lead to a dramatic reduction in flatus formation.
e. Sugar and sugar products also can cause flatulence and can be avoided on the basis of elimination diet.
f. Rice is rarely flatulogenic because its lack of protein binding helps its degradation in the small intestine. However, most other grains (oat, bran, bajra, and wheat) produce moderate flatulence.

Q 33. What are the medicines that can be used to treat gas problem or flatulence?

Many medicines can be used to treat flatulence with varying amount of success. In some cases multiple drugs can be used. These medicines and their mode of actions are as follows:

a. **Carminatives:** These are drugs which give immediate relief to belching and empty the stomach gases. They give a great comfort when the gases get stored in the stomach and lead to fullness of the abdomen. Various drugs used for this purpose are Sodium bicarbonate, peppermint oil, cardamom, oil of dil, tincture ginger (commercial preparations are: Apicarmin syrup, Carmicide syrup, Giger C, Pudin hara, Satya jiban)

b. **Activated Charcoal:** Charcoal tablets are available in the market which may reduce hydrogen and hydrogen sulphide gases by binding with these gases and absorping them. Two tablets can be taken 30 minutes before meals.

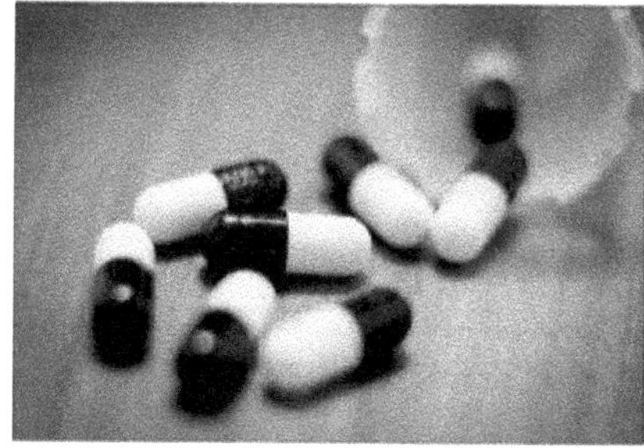

c. **Methyl Polysiloxanes:** Simithicon, dimethicone, dimethyl polysiloxane are some of the drugs which is a silicon polymer that changes the elasticity of the gas bubbles, making them to coalesce or burst. These medicines are often combined with antacids like calcium, magnesium and aluminium hydroxide giving a great relief from flatulence. Hundreds of commercial preparations are available e.g. Dimol, Gelucil MPS, Digene, Diovol, Alcid, Alphagel, Gas pass, Gastrocid, Mintacid, Gasogen,Riflux and so on.

d. **Alpha Galactosidase:** This is an enzyme derived from Aspergillus niger. It decreases bacterial fermentation by degrading oligosaccharides, found in beans, vegetables, cereals to simple sugars especially galactose. It is available both in syrup form and tablet form. Five to fifteen drops of syrup with the first bite of food or 2-3 tablets can be taken with food.Commercial preparations are Baleno syrup, Leno syrup,Tab Biotamax, Tab Geridys, Tab Gaseade.

e. **Digestive Enzyme preparations:** Hundreds of medicines which have enzymes to break down undigested carbohydrates, proteins and fats are available. Pancreatin is a very popular enzyme preparation as it contains amylase, trypsin and lipase. Some of the enzymes are derived from fungus. These can reduce gas formation in the intestine to a great extent. Some of the commercial preparations are Pankreoflat, Unienzyme, Rivozyme, Tonozyme, Peptine, Festal N, Enzar, Gaskit, Arystozyme, Bestozyme. These tablets are prescribed mostly after food.

f. **Treatment of Infections and different types of Colitis:** Amebiasis(infection with the common germ Entamiba hystolytica), Giardiasis(infectctions with Giardia lambia) are two very common germ induced infections called Colitis.Tablets called Metronidazole, Fluroquinolones for 5-7 days often give relief to flatulence. Commercial preparations can be Entamizole, Flagyl, Furoxone, Metrogyl, Dyrade M. If we suspect bacterial infections Tetracyclines, Norfloxacillins, Ciprofloxacillins can also be given to a great relief from gas problem. Combinations of both the drugs are also very effective in many cases. Commercial preparations are Norflox TZ, Ciplox TZ.

g. **Isobgol husk:** It is a non starch poly saccaharide fiber that helps to regulate bowel movements. This can be helpful in case of IBS(Irritable Bowel Syndrome). It is a bulk former and can cause additional flatulence in the first week of use. However this decreases over time and the patients have less flatulence as their bowel habits become regular.

h. **Metclopropamide,** which regulates the bowel movements can also be used in case of flatulence effectively.

Q 34. What are the treatment of Flatulence or Gas by Naturopathy or Yoga?

These include some asanas, Kunjal, Sankhprakshalan. Fasting is also advised in naturopathy where only fruit juices are provided.

Q35. What asanas can be useful in Gas or Flatulence?

BOAT POSE

Perform the Boat Pose to strengthen your abdominal area and hip flexor, tone muscles in the midsection, improve digestion, and relieve stress. You can use a Yoga Strap to aid you in holding the pose longer or if you cannot keep your legs straight.

BOW POSE

The alternating stretching and releasing of the abdominal muscles increases blood flow to this area and aids all sorts of digestive disorders and discomforts. The Bow works all parts of your back simultaneously. The pose is so named because as you hold it, your body is bent back like a bow.

This is simply the easiest of the yoga poses for anxiety. Lie flat on stomach rest your palms besides your shoulders. Holding the feet together and toes pointing away, push-up your head and chest gently off the ground with head lifted up fully. Breathing sequence is inhaling while pushing up and exhaling on the way back.

PIGEON POSE

The Pigeon Pose isolates various muscles in the hips, reducing stiffness and increasing flexibility. It is this isolation of muscles that can make this pose so challenging. Be aware that there is definitely some physical work involved with the practice of this asana. The key is to bring your attention to and observe the sensations created in your body during your practice.

PAVANMUKTASANA

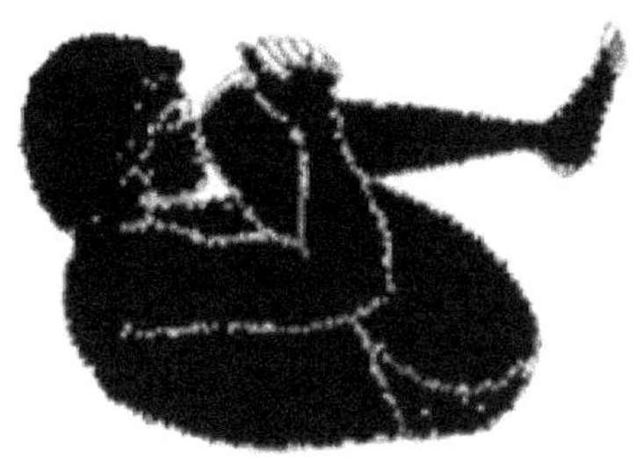

Pavanmuktasana means freedom from air which is related to gaseous distention of stomach and as the name suggests it is beneficial in gas related problems of the stomach. It is also very much useful for persons with spinal problems such as chronic backache, slip disc or sciatica.

Steps

- Lie down on your back, fold your right leg upto the knee and lift the right knee to the chest. Interlock both the hands and keeping them on knee support knee to rest on the chest. Then lift your head and try to touch the knees by your nose. Now hold your breath and remain in this position for 10-20 seconds and then make your leg straight.

- In second stage of Pavanmuktasana both knees should be folded in the same way and the head should be lifted to touch in between the knees by nose as shown in picture below.
- The position of pavanmuktasana should be holded for 10-20 seconds and the entire procedure should be repeated 2-4 times, then second phase of Pavanmuktasana should be done. Complete cycle should then be repeated 3-4 times.

HALASANA

Halasana makes the spine flexible. Halasana improves the strength of the muscles and nerves of the spine. Blood circulation to the neck is increased. The waist becomes free from excess fat. The stomach is pressed well and the abdominal viscera improve their function. Digestion is improved. Constipation is removed. Practice of Halasana slims the body.

Steps

- Lie flat on your back with legs and feet together, arms at the sides, closed and placed beside the thighs.

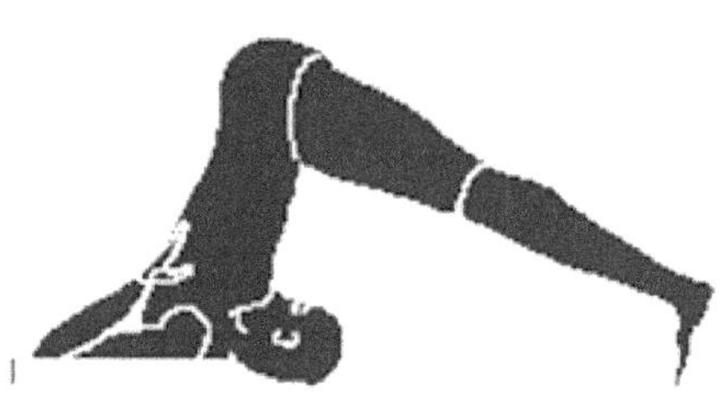

- Keeping your legs straight, inhale slowly, and raise your legs to 30, 60 and 90, pausing at each stage. While exhaling push your legs further over and above the head and then beyond, so that they touch the floor (without bending the knees).
- Stretch your legs as far as possible so that your chin presses tightly against the chest. Then raise your hands and try to hold the toes. Retain the pose from 10 seconds to three minutes. Breathe normally.
- While exhaling, return to the standing position. Slowly go through the process in the reverse order.

DHANURASANA

This asana helps to relieve arthritis and rheumatism. It strengthens the whole body, particularly the lungs, abdominal organs, sciatic nerves, prostate glands and the kidneys. It also provides relief in cases of diabetes, constipation, dyspepsia, bronchitis, etc.

Steps

- Lie down with face and the forehead touching the ground, arms extended alongside the body and legs straight.
- Bend your legs at the knees towards the hips, bringing them forward so that they can be held firmly by the hands at the ankles on the respective sides.
- While inhaling, stretch your legs backwards and raise your thighs, chest and head simultaneously. Hands should be kept straight. The weight of the body should be on the navel. Knees should be kept close, if possible, with eyes looking upwards. This posture should be retained for at least a few seconds, holding the breath.

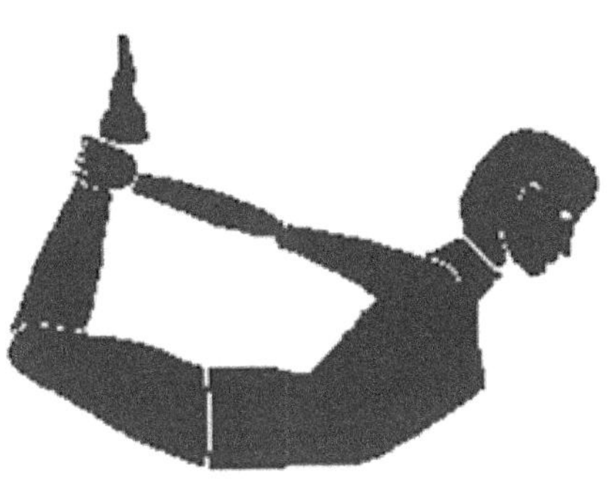

BHUJANGASANA

Bhujangasana is one of the most important Yoga poses. Bhujangasana is also called by the name of Cobra pose. Begin inhaling and raise your chest and head slowly to the maximum limit it can reach. While performing the exercise remember to keep your hip muscles tight so that your lower back is not injured.

Steps

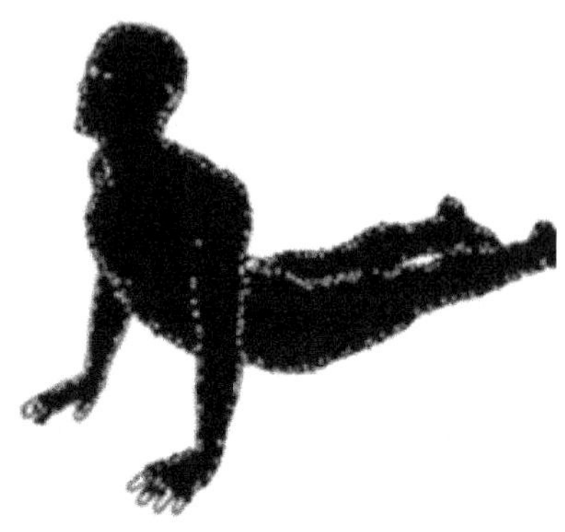

- Lie in the prone position with the forehead resting on the floor, legs straight and feet together, toes pointing backwards, arms bent at the elbows, palms flat on the floor, shoulders and arms on the sides of the chest and fingers kept straight and together.
- Inhale slowly and raise the upper body (head, neck and chest). Look at the ceiling (sky) with the neck bent as far back as possible. For raising the body, only the back muscles are to be used.
- Do not push up with your arms. Waist, legs and toes should remain on the ground. Raise your body as much as possible, holding the position and retaining the breath for a few seconds.
- Exhaling slowly, return to the original position. Repeat three to four times.

Q36. What is Shankha Prakshalan and how does it help?

Shankha Prakshalan is one of the cleansing techniques in yoga which cleanses the entire intestinal tract and detoxifies you completely. This is also quite easy to practice and can be done at home also, but it is important to practice the first time under the guidance of some knowledgeable person. Shankha Prakshala is part of six yogic cleansing practices.

In Shankha Prakshalan, there are 5 poses which are practiced one after another. One cycle consists of the five poses:

1. Tadasana
2. Trivak Tadasana
3. Katichakrasana
4. Trivak Bhujangasana
5. Udarakarshana

> The colon present in the large intestine is a tube stretched from the end of the small intestine through the rectum.

Total of eight rounds or more can be practiced. Between each two rounds two glasses of slightly warm saline water is taken. In between if there is urge to go to the toilet you should go and relieve yourself.

When you go to the toilet the first time the feces will be more solid in nature and as you drink water and complete the entire practice only water would be expelled.

Practice of Shankha Prakshalan helps in eliminating all toxic elements from the body. It has extremely beneficial effect on cough, asthma, helps in losing weight, constipation, migraine and other diseases. This can be practiced once every 6-12 weeks but it should only be practiced under the guidance of some expert.

Q 37. What is Kunjal ?

Kunjal is one of the most effective yogic techniques. It is dramatic and instantaneous in its action. It can give immediate relief to asthmatics and to those suffering from acidity, indigestion, headache, etc. You only need to try it for yourself to find out how effective it is. Kunjal is performed by drinking tepid, salty water up to the point where you feel like vomiting. The water should be lukewarm, and contain about one or two teaspoons of salt for half a litre of water. At least six glasses of water should be drunk, but if you can, drink more -up to the point where you cannot take even one more sip. At this point you may vomit automatically, if not then put two fingers down your throat and massage the back of your tongue as far down as possible. By pressing it you will feel the urge to vomit, which is called the 'gag reflex' in medical terminology. Water will come out of your mouth in a quick series of gushes. Continue pressing until your stomach is empty.

> The liver is the largest gland in the body and is situated in the upper right part of abdominal cavity immediately below the diaphragm in right hypochondriac, epigastric and part of left hypochondriac regions. Its average weight is 1.5 kg.

This practice should be done first thing in the morning on an empty stomach. It is also done after shankhaprakshalana. Follow kunjal with neti.

After completion of the practice, it is best to wait twenty minutes or half an hour before eating. The stomach lining should have a chance to reform before the process of digestion starts pouring acids onto its sensitive surface.

At the physical level, kunjal can aid the maintenance of good health as well as help in the cure of the following diseases: acidity and gas in the stomach; biliousness, nausea, food poisoning and auto-poisoning; indigestion; inflamed oesophageal mucosa, coughs, asthma, bronchitis and respiratory ailments; headaches, (both tension and migraine) and diseases of the nervous system.

Chapter - 3

Acidity & Peptic Ulcer Disease

Q 38. What is Dyspepsia ?

Dyspepsia or Upper abdominal pain is a very common complaint and is caused by a variety of common gastro intestinal diseases – ranging from mild infection of the stomach to serious disease like perforation of the peptic ulcer. Dyspepsia may be a described as stomach ache, cramps, spasms in the upper part of the abdomen. Almost all the people must have experienced such a pain almost once in their life. About 25% people have experienced it in the last one year according to medical statistics.

Q 39. What are the common causes of Upper Abdominal Pain or Dyspepsia?

The most common causes of Dyspepsia are

a. Peptic ulcer – Gastric or Duodenal Ulcer

b. GERD or Gastro Esophageal Reflux Disease

c. Gastritis

Ninety percent of the chronic or prolonged dyspepsia are due to either of the three causes. All three are very common diseases of the gastrointestinal tract. Sometimes or often there may not be any reason of short lived dyspepsia - these are then called Non Ulcer Dyspepsia.

Q40. What are the uncommon causes of Upper Abdominal Pain?

a. Stones in the gall bladder
b. Pancreatitis
c. Pancreatic and gastric cancer
d. Perforated duodenal ulcer
e. Some cases of Heart attack
f. Bursting of the aorta in the abdomen

Q 41. What are the common associated complaints with Upper Abdominal Pain?

Common associated symptoms may be heartburn, fullness of the abdomen, Nausea, vomiting, hiccup or belching. Loss of appetite, acute cramps may also be there in some cases.

Q 42. What is PEPTIC ULCER ?

Peptic ulcer is one of the most serious diseases of the gastrointestinal tract, particularly the stomach. The prevalence of ulcers has been increasing over the past few years owing to rapid changes in the dietary habits and lifestyle practices.

The term peptic ulcer is used to describe any localized erosion of the lining of that portion of the alimentary tract that comes in contact with acidic stomach juice. The destruction of tissues can also result in necrosis. The majority of ulcers are found in the duodenum – the area just after the stomach, although they also occur in the oesophagus, stomach or jejunum. Similar symptoms are produced by the ulcer regardless of its location and response to treatment is essentially the same.

Q 43. How these ulcers are formed?

Acids are present in the stomach and help to digest the food. Another chemical called Pepsin is also produced by the stomach to break down the food particles. Both these have capacity to digest or destroy the stomach wall.

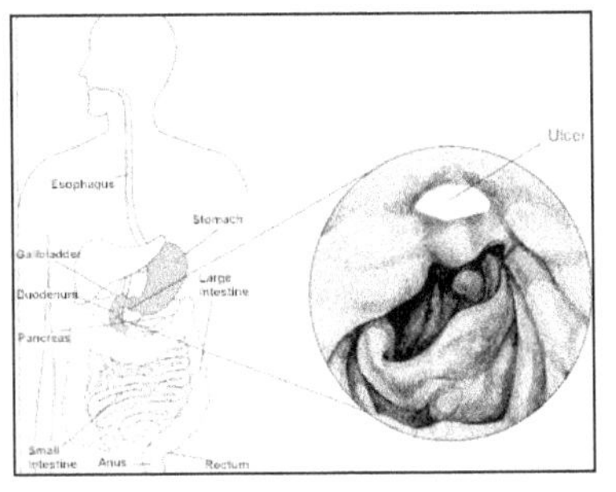

The three vital mechanisms that protect the stomach walls are the mucous layer, prostaglandins and probably the urogastrone/ epidermal healing factor (URO/EHF).These mechanisms can protect the stomach against hydrochloric acid up to twice the maximum concentration which the stomach is capable of secreting.

The mucous layer, viscous gel ideally situated for its function of protection from chemical and physical hazards of waterproofing and lubrication. This mucous is secreted by the mucous cells present in the glands present in the wall of the stomach. The gastric mucosa also secretes bicarbonate which combines with the mucous and form this mucous coat which protect the stomach walls from the action of the acids.

The second line of defense is prostaglandins. They are released locally in the mucosa and sub mucosa in response to any irritant stimulus. They instantly accelerate cell replacement, opening up the microcirculation to bring cell nutrients and to remove toxic metabolites. It is a mechanism which enables the gastric mucosa to withstand even absolute alcohol and boiling water and to counter a wide variety of chemical hazards even without any help from simultaneous reduction of gastric acid secretion. Their efficiency probably also depends on there being an adequate dietary supply of essential fatty acids for their formation.

Urogastrone (third line of defense) plays an important role by inhibiting gastric acid secretion on the one hand and by stimulation of cell proliferation and regeneration on the other and healing ulcer.

Usually there is a balance between acid, pepsin secretion and mucosal resistance. For reasons that we still do not understand well this balance is disturbed. As a result of excess acid production or weakening in the integrity of the stomach membrane or both, the mucosal lining is broken and the underlying layers of the stomach are exposed to the effect of the concentrated acid resulting in peptic ulcer.

Q 44. What is this mucus and how do they protect stomach?

When someone coughs, you will see sometime the cough has a water coloured thick jelly. This is the secretion of the mucosal cells in the breathing tubes. Such mucosal or mucous producing cells are also present in the stomach wall. They keep on producing such thick jelly type sticky material and form a layer of this thick jelly all over the stomach wall. Thus, the mucous layer do not allow the acid and pepsin to digest the stomach wall and cause peptic ulcer.

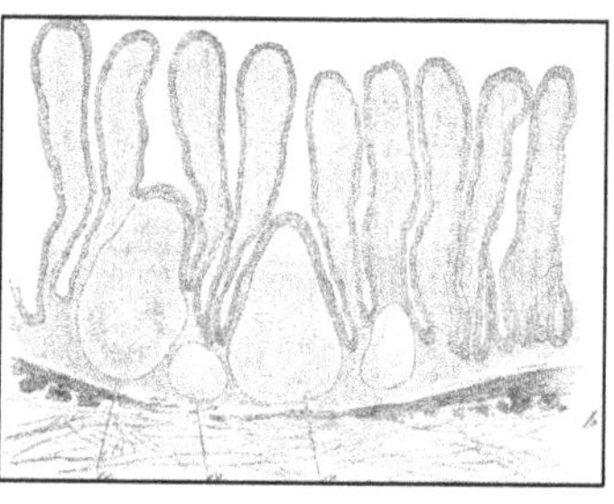

The factors that influence mucosal ability to withstand destructive action are

- The integrity of mucosal cells
- The ability of epithelial cells to regenerate themselves
- The mucosal barrier
- The blood supply

Various topical irritants impair this protective mucous lining, including aspirin, alcohol, certain drugs, caffeine or bile acids that may come in contact with the mucosa.

Q 45. How the acids are formed inside the stomach and what is the function of this acid?

The acid secreted by the stomach wall is Hydrochloric acid(HCl). In the body and fundus of the stomach, there are parietal cells which produce this acid. The main source of Hydrogen is from water break down. Chlorine is obtained by exchange of carbonic acid in these cells. There is a proton pump mechanism which help in the formation of the acid. This acid produced kills germs in the stomach wall, break down the proteins, brings down the pH of the stomach so that the protein enzyme pepsin can act. The acid also stimulates the secretion of the bile from the liver and pancreatic juice from the pancreas.

Q 46. Can the stomach walls produce more acid ?

More acid can be produced by the stomach by Histamine, Acetyl Choline, and Gastrin. These three act by some proteins called the receptors. Histamine works through H2 receptors. Nerve stimulation releases Acetyle Choline which act through M1 muscarine receptors and Gastrin acts by stimulating Gastrin receptors. Gastrin is a hormone and reaches stomach through blood. Presence of food in the mouth also stimulates the production of acid in the stomach. Psychic stress helps to release gastrin and then the acid secretion. Anger and hostility also produce more acid in the stomach.

Q 47. What is Duodenal ulcer?

Duodenum is the first few inches of the small intestine at

the stomach end. The wall of the duodenum does not have that much protection as the stomach wall against acid. So, if there is excess acid in the stomach content passing out from stomach to duodenum – the wall of the duodenum gets burned by the acid and ulcer is formed. This may be called hyperacidity. Even rapid emptying of the stomach can also lead to such ulcers – as the time required to neutralize the acid is not available.

Q 48. What is Gastric ulcer?

If the peptic ulcer occurs in the stomach wall – it is called gastric ulcer. Most important cause of such ulcers is decreased protection of the stomach walls by the acid resistant mucus layer. This may occur due to less blood supply to the mucous glands present in the stomach wall. Also there is a mechanism that reduce the acid and pepsin production in the stomach – if that system fail more acid and pepsin can also damage the gastric/ stomach wall leading to gastric ulcer.

(Factors that contribute to weaken mucosal resistance in patients with gastric ulcer revolve around poor nutrition, diminished mucosal blood flow and a defect in the inhibition of gastric acid and pepsin secretion.)

> Every day the liver produces about a litre (1.76 pints) of bile. Although over 95% water, it contains a wide range of chemicals including bile salts, mineral salts, cholesterol and bile pigments which give the bile its own characteristic and colour.

In gastric ulcer, both the back diffusion of hydrogen ions into the mucosa and reflux of bile are believed to be involved. An abnormality in the mucosa permits penetrations of hydrogen ions. Drugs such as aspirin and indomethiacin (used in rheumatoid arthritis) can alter the gastric mucosal barrier. Reflux of bile acids from the duodenum due to an incompetent pyloric sphincter leads to chronic gastritis and subsequent ulceration. Gastric ulcers are more prone to develop into malignant disease.

In the development of gastric ulcers although the presence of acid is essential, the degree of tissue sensitivity seems to be the paramount factor. In the patient with duodenal ulcer, excess production of acid and pepsin is the primary factor.

Q 49. Normally the ulcers do not form in the stomach or Duodenum. What are the factors that help in formation of such ulcers?

a. Bacterial infection: Helicobacter pyroli is the chief cause of ulcer. It is spiral shaped, unipolar flagellum and is associated with antral gastritis and duodenitis in the presence of gastric metaplasia. H.pyroli infection is strongly implicated which has a damaging effect on the mucosal defense thereby increasing the vulnerability to ulceration.

b. Genetic factor: It is common in persons with blood group O than in those of other groups and possibly in those with HLA-B5 antigens. People who are first degree relatives of patients with duodenal ulcer have an increased risk of developing duodenal ulcer.

c. Sex: Men are affected two to three times more frequently than women.

d. Age: The incidence is high between 20 and 40 though the average age of incidence has increased. During these years, career and personal striving are at a peak.

e. Stress: People who are highly nervous and emotional and who worry, fear and feel anxiety are particularly susceptible. This emotional and nervous control of the vascular system in the gastric or duodenal walls may be so disturbed that there is diminution in the blood supply to the mucosa of the stomach and duodenum making it susceptible to acid secretion.

f. Potentially irritant substances: Caffeine, ethanol, aspirin and nicotine may delay healing but there is little evidence to show that these substances induce ulcer. Chillies, pepper, ginger, garam masala, meat soups and strong tea or coffee and protein rich foods increase the secretion of hydrochloric acid and aggravate the condition.

g. High fiber: In India the incidence of peptic ulcer is low where the staple diet is millet or wheat compared to rice eating area. This theory is yet to be confirmed.

h. Emergency injuries: Stress ulcers occur in conjunction with emergency injuries such as burns or long-term rehabilitation processes.

Q 50. What are the complaints of the patient suffering from Peptic Ulcer (Symptoms and clinical findings)?

The following are the main difficulties that a patient of peptic ulcer will face. One or two of them may be present in some patients but some patients may have all of the following.

- Epigastric pain (upper and middle pain in the abdomen), heart burn etc due to reflux of acid into oesophagus occurring as deep hunger contraction 1 to 3 hours after meals is often the chief complaint. The pain may be described as dull, pierching, burning or gnawing and is usually relieved by the taking food or alkalies.
- Discomfort and flatulence in upper part of abdomen. The basis for the pain may be the action of unneutralised hydrochloric acid on exposed nerve fibres at the site of the ulcer.
- Pain is also associated with hypermotility of the stomach or gastric distention following ingestion of large amounts of food or liquids.
- Low plasma protein levels are often present and delay rapid and complete healing of the ulcer.
- Weight loss and iron deficiency anaemia are common.

- The intake of iron, ascorbic acid and B complex vitamin, particularly thiamine may be less than desirable because of self imposed limitation of leafy green vegetables and other good source of these nutrients.
- In some instances, haemorrhage is the first indication of an ulcer and requires surgical intervention. Other complications such as obstruction, perforation and carcinoma of the gastric ulcer are treated surgically.
- Bleeding ulcers can result in vomiting known as haematemesis (dark brown in colour).
- There are spasms of pyloric canal and this may give rise to a feeling of sickness distension and prevent taking food.

Q51. What are the main cause of Peptic Ulcer?

Two drugs which mostly lead to the ulcer formation are Aspirin (Acetyl salicylic Acid) and pain killer drugs called NSAID (Non Steroidal Anti Inflammatory Drugs). Aspirin is used to prevent clotting of blood in heart patients and patients with paralysis. On prolonged use it can lead to peptic ulcer. NSAID drugs like brufen inhibit the production of prostaglandin which help in mucus production and secrete bicarbonate. Both of them protect ulcer formation.

Another cause of peptic ulcer is supposed to be infection of a germ called Helicobacter pylori which causes inflammation of the stomach wall. This is also one of major suspected factor leading to peptic ulcer.

> Without bile our bodies cannot digest fat. It is made in the liver, stored in the gall bladder and does its work in the small intestines.

Q52. What are the outside factors associated with Peptic Ulcer ?

Factors	Gastric ulcer	Duodenal ulcer
Environmental influences	Cigarette smoking Aspirin, pain killer abuse Alcohol consumption	Cigarette smoking Aspirin, pain killer abuse Alcohol consumption
Associated diseases	Chronic bronchitis and emphysema Antral gastritis (duodenal ulcer in 20%)	Cirrhosis of liver Pancreatic cancer Chronic bronchitis and emphysema Renal stones
Basic pathophysiology	Mainly, lowered mucosal resistance. Acid pepsin levels normal to low, but some acid requiste.	Mainly, excessive acid pepsin secretion, Lowered muscosal resistance may contribute.

Q 53. What may be the complications of Peptic ulcer?

People with ulcers may experience serious complications if they do not get treatment. The most common problem includes – Bleeding from the ulcer, perforation of the wall of the stomach or duodenum and narrowing of the duodenum or last end of the stomach. All the three are very serious complications – if not treated may lead to death as well.

Q.54. What happens when the ulcer starts bleeding?

As an ulcer eats into the muscles of the stomach or duodenal wall, blood vessels may also be damaged, causing bleeding. A bleeding ulcer goes unnoticed for few hours or even a day – and often not detected till the stool becomes black. The blood become black coloured when it reacts with the acid of the stomach. This bleeding ulcer is also seen in heart patients who take aspirin for a long period in presence of an ulcer. Many painkillers, especially anti inflammatory group can also precipitate this ulcer bleeding. The patient feels weakness when the hemoglobin falls after about a litre of blood is lost. Pain in the abdomen may or may not occur with a bleeding ulcer. Death may occur if the bleeding gets unnoticed for longer period.

Q 55. What happens when there is a perforation of the stomach or duodenal wall?

Perforation is the bursting of the stomach wall or duodenal wall due to excess erosion. The ulcer creates a hole in the wall of the stomach or duodenum, and bacteria and partially digested food can spill through the opening into the abdominal cavity (peritoneum) and cause peritonitis an inflammation of the abdominal cavity and wall. This is a very serious condition and usually accompanied by acute abdominal pain, hard abdomen.

Q 56. How narrowing or obstruction occurs in the stomach or duodenum?

If ulcer is located at the end of the stomach, where the duodenum is attached, it can cause swelling and scarring which can narrow or close the intestinal opening. This obstruction can prevent food from leaving the stomach and entering the small intestine, resulting in vomiting the contents of the stomach.

Q 57. What tests can be done to identify Peptic ulcer?

Radiographic examination with Barium Meal: The technique, though simple, carries a fairly substantial risk of missing the problem.

Endoscopy: A flexible tube made of fibre optic bundles introduced into the stomach and the endoscopist inspects the food pipe and stomach and detects any breaks in the lining membrane. It takes 15-20 minutes. If there is cancer, it can also be detected by endoscopy.

Biopsy: A biopsy of lining tissue.

Acid secretion of the stomach: In this, the acid output after stimulation by pentagastrin is measured. It is useful for further investigation if surgery is contemplated. Acid output is higher than normal in duodenal ulcer and low or absent in patients with carcinoma of the stomach.

Q 58. What is the treatment of Stomach or Duodenal Ulcer?

The treatment of peptic ulcer involves mainly three steps – selection of correct food; modification of the eating habits; rest and avoidance of excess stress; and of course, medicines.

Q 59. What are the foods to be avoided and taken as the treatment of Peptic Ulcer?

It was customary to suggest a bland diet for ulcer patients. Bland diet is a diet which is mechanically, chemically and thermally non-irritating.

Mechanically irritating foods include those with indigestible carbohydrate, such as whole grains and most raw fruits and vegetables. Foods believed to be chemically irritating because of their stimulatory effect on gastric secretion include meat extractives, caffeine, alcohol and some spicy foods. The capsaicin present in chillies causes shedding of surface stomach cells and may cause peptic distress. Foods believed to be thermally irritating are those ordinary served at extremes of temperatures, such as very hot or iced liquids may cause pain. This diet prevents irritation to the mucosa, avoids increase in acidity and aids in control of pain.

Sound total nutrition: There must be optimal overall

nutritional intake to support recovery and maintain healthy tissue, based on individual needs and food tolerances.

Protein foods: Milk and protein foods do have some buffering effect but they also evoke gastric secretions more than carbohydrates and fats. Milk should be included as a source of nutrient factors for healing purposes. Protein provides the necessary amino acids for synthesis of tissue protein which helps in healing ulcer.

Fat: Moderate amount of the fat helps to suppress gastric secretion and motility through the enterogastrone mechanism. Fat such as cream, butter and olive oil can be particularly helpful in a thin patient. Fried foods are not advised as they are difficult to digest and often aggravate the symptoms.

Ascorbic acid: It helps in wound healing hence citrus fruit juice and tomato juice can be given. The pH of food before ingestion has little significance.

Gas former: In addition, certain foods traditionally forbidden include strongly flavoured vegetables such as cabbage, cauliflower, onions, turnip and fried foods. Restriction of these foods is based on subjective evidence from patients who experience distress following ingestion of these items.

Fibre: A regular diet, including good food sources of dietary fibre, has proved to be beneficial.

By trial and error patient should decide which foods to be included or avoided. Possible foods that are to be avoided and included are given below:

Foods to be included	Foods to be avoided
Dairy products like milk, cream, butter, cheese and egg (not fried), steamed fish, rice, rice flakes, puffed rice, well-cooked cereals, semolina, cooked green leafy vegetables, custards, malted drinks, cooked pulses (if they are not causing gas formation).	Alcohol, strong tea, coffee, cola beverages, gravies, pickles, spices, chillies, curries, condiments, all fried foods, pastries, cakes, heavy sweets like halwa, barfi, raw unripe fruits, raw vegetables like cucumber, onions, radish and tomatoes.

Management:

What are to be done by

Patient	Doctors	Practice
Put a stop to alcohol and smoking. Control your stress. Restrict the consumption of irritant substances like caffeine, aspirin, nicotine as they delay healing.	Avoid ulcer promoting drugs like pain killers, steroids. Give knowledge and educate the patients. Medicines to prevent and heal the ulcer.	✓ Eat a bland diet ✓ Take a sound total nutrition ✓ Avoid gas forming foods ✓ Regularity of meal time is essential ✓ Have food slowly and chew properly

Q60. What eating habits an ulcer patient should adopt ?

- Whether a patient is on bland diet or regular diet, he needs to know which foods are needed for a nutritionally adequate diet and the importance of including these daily.
- He should select food from a wide variety of foods, omitting those foods known to be distressing to the patient.
- Regularity of mealtimes is essential. The patient gets benefited by small and frequent meals.
- In between meals, protein rich snacks should be taken.
- Moderate amounts of food should be eaten. Heavy meals are avoided. Volume of any foods sufficient to exert antral pressure against the stomach wall stimulates gastric secretion through the gastrin mechanism.
- The diet should be planned in consultation with patient, taking into consideration his preferences, cultural pattern and economic status.
- Meals eaten outside the house will not cause any problem if good judgement is used in food selection.
- A short rest before and after meals may be conductive to

greater enjoyment of meals.

- Food should be eaten slowly and chewed well. How one eats is more important than what one eats because fast eating provokes gastric feeding reflex.

Q 61. Does smoking and alcohol lead to ulcers? What to do about them?

Smoking and drinking alcohol should be avoided particularly on an empty stomach. Smoking causes pyloric incompetence and reflux of duodenal juice into stomach. Smoking also interferes with attempts to decrease gastric acid and pepsin secretion with drugs.

Q 62. How rest and avoidance of excess stress help the ulcer patients?

Good physical and mental health is basic if the person is to learn to cope with his or her problems constructively. Mental and physical rest is important modification of living and work habits is needed when overwork and physical stress cause exacerbations of the disease. The patient should remember that anxiety and worry can upset digestion.

Q63. What are the medicines used to treat peptic ulcer?

The following groups of medicines are commonly used to treat Peptic ulcer. These are;

a. Antacids – these neutralize the acid present in the stomach
b. H2 receptor Antagonists
c. Proton Pump Inhibitors
d. Metoclopramide – dopamine antagonists
e. Drugs for giving pain relief.

Surgical treatments are almost rare after the introduction of the above drugs.

Q64. What are Antacids?

Antacids are alkaline chemicals which can neutralize acids in the stomach and duodenum. They are available in syrup and tablet forms. Most of the antacids have Alluminium hydroxide, Magnesium hydroxide and carbonate and Calcium Carbonate. Sometimes they are added by other chemicals which can coat the ulcers with acid protective silicon compounds.

Some of the popular antacids commercially available are: Digene, Diavol, Gelusil, Sigma, Solacid. They are given as 2-4 tsf two to four times in a day.

Q65. What are the H2 receptor Inhibitor drugs and what do they do?

Stopping of acid secretion or minimizing the acid formation is the main function of the Histamine receptor Antogonists or inhibitors. Thus, the acids cannot erode the walls of the stomach or duodenum and ulcers can heal comfortably. Four groups of H2 receptor Antagonists are very popular and widely available – Cimetidine, famotidine, Nizatidine and Ranitidine. They are more effective in reducing night-time acid secretion and used more during sleep time. The usual doses of cimetidine is 400mg BD, famotidine is 20mg BD, Nizatidine is 150mg BD and Ranitidine is 150mg BD. Most of these medicines have no major side effects and can be taken in long term.

Some of the popular commercial preparations of this group of medicines are as follows:

Cimetidine: Cimetidine, Tymidin, Ulciban

Ranitidine: Aciloc, Histac, Ranicure, Ranitidine,Ranitine, Rantac, Zinetac

Famotidine: Famtac, Acipep, Topcid, Famocid.

Roxatidine: Rotane, Zorpex.

Q66. What are the Proton Pump Inhibitors and what do they do?

These drugs block the Proton Pump present in the cells in the stomach wall which secrete acid. Their effects on the gastric acid production is much more as compared to the H2 receptor Antagonists and can decrease the acid production by almost 90%. The major groups of Proton Pump Inhibitors are Omeprazole, Lansoprazole, Rebeprazole, Pantoprazole and Esomaprazole. The usual doses are Omeprazole 20mg BD, Lansoprazole 15mg BD, Rebeprazole 20mg BD, Pantoprazole 40mg BD and Esomaprazole 20mg BD. They can be used four times a day also.

Some of the popular commercial preparations of this group of medicines are as follows:

Omeprazole: Omez, Oprazole, Acicure, Om, Nucid

Lansoprazole: Lan, Lancus, Lansol, Lona

Pantoprazole: Pan, Pancop 40, Pantocid, Pantodac,Pfd

Rapeprazole: Happi, Mosarab, Nucid, Cyra, Rabegon

Esomeprazole: Espra, Esoz, Sompraz

Q67. What are Metoclopramides drugs and what do they do?

Metoclopramides are drugs which promote esophageal movements and emptying of the stomach. They also improve the sphincter present at the lower end of the esophagus. They are called prokinetic drugs. Some of the drugs commercially available preparations of this group are: Perinorm, Reglan, Periglo.

Q 68. Recently peptic ulcer is also said to be due to a germ called Helicobacter pylori. Is it true? How to treat this infection?

Though not very clear but infection of the stomach by this bacteria is supposed to cause or aggravate ulcer formation. To treat this infection a combination of four drugs are used for a period of 14 days. These are Tetracycline, Metronidazole, Bismuth and Lansoprazole. This treatment is also useful in gastritis patients.

Chapter - 4

Heartburn or Acid Reflux (GERD)

Q 69. What is heartburn ?

It is a sense of burning felt below the central bone of the chest (called Sternum). It usually radiates towards the mouth or throat – specially after heavy meals during weight lifting, bending over or just lying flat. This problem is very common and affects crores (ten millions) of people.

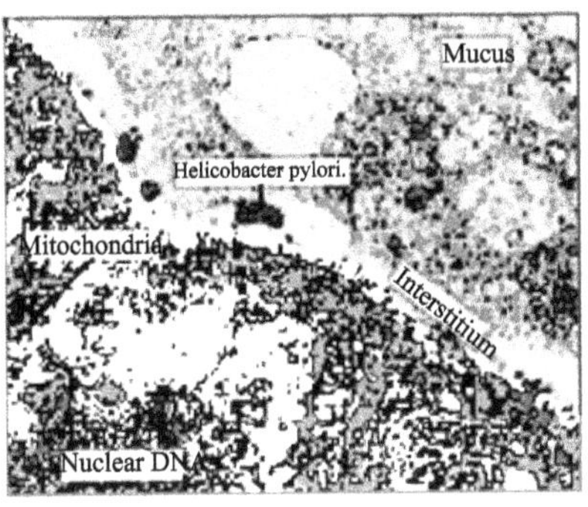

Q 70. What are the most common causes of heartburn?

The most common cause of heartburn is a disease called GERD (Gastro Esophageal Reflux Disease). Reflux or regurgitation or back flow of the stomach contents occur in this disease. This acid burns the unprotected wall of the esophagus – leading to pain under the breastbone.

The second most cause of heartburn is heart attack. The other causes may be disease of the esophagus (Esophageal inflammation, excessive movement or hypermotility, hypersensitive esophageal door or sphincter). Some of the lung diseases can also lead to symptoms of heartburn.

Q 71. What are the accompanying symptoms of Heartburn?

Heart burn is often associated with nausea, dyspepsia(upper abdominal pain), bloating (fullness of the abdomen), belching and indigestion. Many people get up in the night due to such acute pain from GERD. Water brush – sudden filling up of the mouth with bitter or salty fluid can also happen with heartburn.

Q 72. Are there any common precipitating factors leading to heartburn?

Large meals, spicy food, citrus foods, high fat meals, colas, coffee, teas usually proceed heartburn condition. Meals close to the bedtime, beers and alcohol with meals increase night-time symptoms of heart burn.

Q73. How to distinguish between Heart pain and acid regurgitation pain?

Most of the heart pain or angina pain occurs on the left side of the chest. They have a relation with exertion – they increase with walking and reduce on taking rest. During heart attack, only the pain in the chest occurs at rest. But mostly this pain occurs on the left side of the chest, radiating to the left arm.

Only in a small percentage of heart attacks, the pain may be in the center of the chest and may be mistaken as heart burn. Heart pain can come any time when the heart attack comes but substernal pain occurring with or after meals point towards esophageal heartburn. If the pain occurs in lying down position, lasting for more than one hour, leads to awakening of the patient from sleep it suggests esophageal pain. The esophageal pain usually gets relieved by just sitting up within few minutes – heart pain will not.

Relief of pain by antacids also suggest heart burn. Taking a tablet of sorbitrate below the tongue also relieves pain of spasm of esophageal sphincter and can give a false alarm of heart pain. Heart pain as rest should be taken as heart attack and should be excluded by ECG and Troponin I test (a slide test where a drop of blood can diagnose heart attack in a minute).

Q 74. What is GERD?

When we swallow food it passes through a 40cm long food pipe called Esophagus and the food reaches the stomach at the end of this food pipe. There is a muscular door (called Sphincter or lower esophageal sphincter or LES) at the junction of the esophagus and stomach which allows food to pass to the stomach but prevents the contents of the stomach (gastric cavity) to return back to the esophagus. This back flow of the food to the esophagus is called reflux or regurgitation. This disease is called GERD or Gastro Esophageal Reflux Disease.

Q 75. What is Regurgitation?

Regurgitation (or reflux) is defined as the effortless return of the gastric contents into the esophagus and more frequently into the mouth. There is a distinct feeling of acid or bitter taste in the chest or mouth with regurgitation.

This is a very common problem is different from Vomiting – which is mostly voluntary. Regurgitation does not have any symptom of nausea or vomiting sensation.

> Bile salts return to the liver in the blood of the portal vein, twice during the process of digestion.

Q76. What is the problem if the contents of the stomach regurgitates to the esophagus?

The gastric or Stomach contents have a good concentration of acid in it. But this acid cannot burn the stomach wall as they are protected by a layer of mucous. But the wall of the esophagus does not have this protection. So, the acid burns the lower end of the food pipe or esophagus – leading to this heart burn condition.

Q77. Give us some more details on GERD.

Gastro Esophageal Reflux Disease, commonly referred to as GERD or acid reflux, is a condition in which the liquid content of the stomach regurgitates (backs up or refluxes) into the esophagus. The liquid can inflame and damage the lining (cause esophagitis) of the esophagus although visible signs of inflammation occur in a minority of patients. The regurgitated liquid usually contains acid and pepsin that are produced by the stomach. (Pepsin is an enzyme that begins the digestion of proteins in the stomach.) The refluxed liquid also may contain bile that has backed-up into the stomach from the duodenum. (The duodenum is the first part of the small intestine that attaches to the stomach.) Acid is believed to be the most injurious component of the refluxed liquid. Pepsin and bile also may injure the esophagus, but their role in the production of esophageal inflammation and damage is not as clear as the role of acid.

GERD is a chronic condition. Once it begins, it usually lasts for longer time. If there is injury to the lining of the esophagus (esophagitis), this also is a chronic condition. Moreover, after the esophagus has healed with treatment and treatment is stopped, the injury will return in most patients within a few months begun, therefore, it usually will need to be continued indefinitely although it is argued that in some patients with intermittent symptoms and no esophagitis, treatment can be intermittent and done only during symptomatic periods.

Gastroesophageal reflux disease or GERD, is a very common disorder and occurs when stomach acid refluxes into the lower esophagus through the lower esophageal sphincter (LES). The LES is a band of muscles that act as a protective barrier against reflux material by contracting and relaxing. If this barrier is relaxed at inappropriate times or otherwise compromised, reflux occurs. Chronic or reoccurring reflux allows prolonged contact of stomach contents with the lower esophagus, leading to the symptoms of GERD. In general, there are four underlying conditions that are associated with GERD:

1. Decreased lower esophageal sphincter pressure.
2. Irritation of the lining of the esophagus by the stomach contents.
3. Abnormal clearance of esophageal acid.
4. Delayed stomach emptying.

Q78. What is Hiatus Hernia?

A Hiatus Hernia or Hiatal Hernia may also contribute to acid reflux. A Hiatal Hernia occurs when the upper part of the stomach is above the diaphragm, the muscle wall that separates the stomach from the chest. The diaphragm helps the LES keep acid from coming up into the esophagus. When a Hiatal Hernia is present, it is easier for the acid to come up. In this way, a Hiatal Hernia can cause reflux. A Hiatal Hernia can happen in people of any age; many otherwise healthy people over 50 have a small one.

> Biles gets its colour from the presence of a pigment called bilirubin. One of the many jobs of the liver is to break down worn out red blood cells.

Other factors that may contribute to GERD include alcohol use, overweight, pregnancy and smoking. Also, certain foods can be associated with reflux events, including citrus fruits, chocolate, drinks with caffeine, fatty and fried foods, garlic and onions, mint flavorings, spicy foods, tomato-based foods like spaghetti sauce, chili, and pizza.

Q 79. What are the symptoms associated with GERD?

GERD is characterized by symptoms and/or tissue damage that result from repeated or prolonged exposure of the lining of the esophagus to the acidic contents of the stomach. The primary symptom of GERD is persistent heartburn, a burning discomfort felt in the upper chest or abdomen and nausea after eating. Symptoms of GERD, however, vary from person to person and at times, there may be no symptoms at all. The majority of people with GERD have mild symptoms, with no visible evidence of tissue damage and little risk of developing complications.

Q 80. What are the complications of GERD?

The possible complications of GERD are esophageal erosion, esophageal ulcer, and esophageal stricture, replacement of the normal esophageal epithelium with abnormal (Barrett's) epithelium and pulmonary aspiration.

Q 81. What are the ways to diagnose GERD?

The possible investigations for GERD may the as follows:

a. Endoscopy of the esophagus and stomach
b. Prolonged pH monitoring
c. Barium meal test for esophagus
d. Provocation by acid and see the results
e. Checking esophageal pressure
f. Therapeutic trial: Treating the GERD by Omeprazole and seeing the pH of the esophagus

Q 82. What is endoscopy ? Is it a sure shot test?

In endoscopy, the patient is asked to swallow a fiber optic tube and light and camera and then it can be pushed to the lower end of the esophagus or food pipe. Since the doctors give a local anaesthetic drug in the throat before endoscopy – swallowing becomes possible.

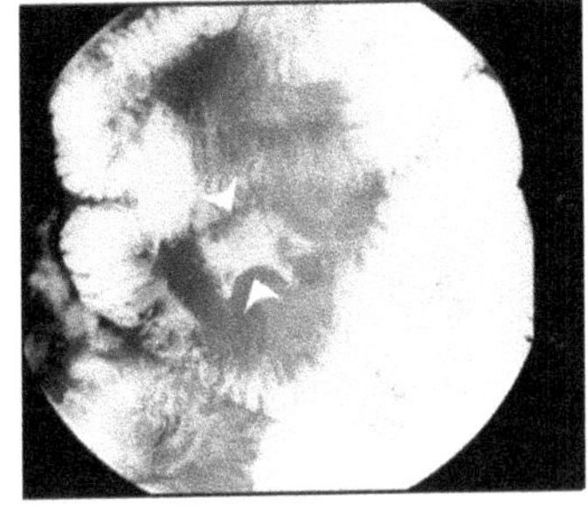

In GERD, endoscopy mostly show inflation of the lower esophageal end or erosion. This is due to acid digestion of the area. It can also show the severity of the disease and also predict how long the treatment should be carried on. Endoscopy should be definitely done if the patient has difficulty in eating, weight loss or bleeding through mouth.

Q 83. What is pH monitoring?

When we want to know any liquid is acidic or alkaline pH is measured. Neutral food has a pH of 7, acidic liquid will have lower pH like 3,4,5,6 and alkaline fluid is 8, 9 etc. In this case miniature pH electrodes are placed and the pH is recorded in the computer for a prolonged time like 24 hours. It can detect the acid in the lower end of the esophagus and tell us about its relation with food and also the results after taking medicines.

Q 84. What is barium meal study and what is expected?

Barium meal study is easy and need a series of X rays after swallowing Barium liquid.This facility is available in small towns also. This can diagnose Haitus Hernia, stricture(permanent contraction) of the lower end of Esophagus, esophageal ring.

Q. 85. What is a provocative test for GERD?

In this test low concentration on Hydrochloric acid is injected in the food pipe to reproduce the heart burn or symptoms reported by the patient. This is followed by the same test with normal saline introduction – which should not produce any symptoms. This test is called Bernstein test.

Q 86. What is esophageal manometry?

This measures the pressure of the lower end of the esophagus and indicated in case the patient plans a surgical treatment of LES (Lower Esophageal Sphincter).

Q87. What is this therapeutic trial?

This is a very interesting test where drugs are given to the patient which are known to reduce the acid secretion in the stomach for one week to ten days. If there is a 75% reduction in the symptoms – the heartburn disappears – the test is positive. Omeprazole 40mg two times a day or Ranitidine 150mg twice a day is mostly used. These drugs can be also used for 8 weeks.

Q 88. What are the treatment options of GERD?

There are four goals in the treatment of the GERD – these are:

a. Reduction of the symptoms or pain or heart burn
b. Healing of the erosion or esophagitis
c. Management and/ or prevention of complications
d. Maintenance of the relief stage for a long period.

Q89. What measures can be taken to alleviate the symptoms?

Diet content modification, alteration of the diet habits, avoidance of drugs which promote acid formation, use of antacids(which neutralize the acid) and drugs which reduce the production of excess acid in the stomach (H2 receptor antagonists and proton pump inhibitors) are the main stream treatment for relief or symptoms. These drugs also help to heal the erosion or inflammation.

Q90. What are the Diet modifications recommended for relief from heart burn or acid reflux?

Dietary modifications are recommended to lessen the likelihood of reflux and to avoid irritation of sensitive or inflamed esophageal tissue. Listed below are several recommendations that may help to manage GERD:

Decrease total fat intake - High fat meals and fried foods tend to decrease LES pressure and delay stomach emptying thereby increasing the risk of reflux.

Avoid large meals - Large meals increase the likelihood of increased gastric (stomach) pressure and reflux.

Decrease total caloric intake if weight loss is desired - Since obesity may promote reflux, weight loss may be suggested by your healthcare provider to control reflux. Reducing both total fat and caloric intake will aid in weight loss.

Avoid chocolate - Chocolate contains methylxanthine, which has been shown to reduce LES pressure by causing relaxation of smooth muscle.

Avoid coffee depending on individual tolerance - Coffee, with or without caffeine, may promote gastroesophageal reflux. Coffee may be consumed if it is well tolerated.

Avoid other known irritants - Alcohol, mint, carbonated beverages, citrus juices, and tomato products all may aggravate GERD. These products may be consumed depending on individual tolerance.

Q 91. What are the habit modifications for treatment of reflux acidity or heartburn?

These are as follows:

- Maintain upright posture during and after eating.
- Stop smoking.
- Avoid clothing that is tight in the abdominal area.
- Avoid eating within 3 hours before bedtime.
- Lose weight if you are overweight.
- Sleep on your left side. This produces less esophageal acid exposure than lying on the right.
- Chew non-mint gum that will increase saliva production and decrease acid in the esophagus.
- Elevate the head of your bed 4-6 inches by placing bricks under the headboard. Instead, 6 to 7 Pillows can be used to raise the head end of the patient during sleep. Hospital beds where the head end of the bed can be raised can also be used to a great relief to the patient.

Q92. What are the medicines used for treatment of GERD or acid reflux?

These fall into four categories:

a. Antacids – liquid or tablet form

b. H2 receptor blocker drugs like Ranitidine

c. Proton pump inhibitors like Pantaprazoles

d. Promotility drugs like metoclopramides

Q93. What are the drugs and dosage of the Antacids?

Most of the antacids contain Calcium Carbonate, Aluminium hydroxide, Magnesium carbonate/Hydroxide/Trisilicate and Magaldrate. These are alkaline substances that neutralize the gastric acid and lead to rise in the pH of stomach. This helps the ulcers to heal. These antacids do not reduce the production of the acid. Some of the antacid also have local anaesthetic agent to reduce gastric pain (Mucaine Gel). They are available more commonly in syrup form but tablets are also available. Some of the popular commercial preparations are – Digene, Diavol, Gelusil, Sigma, Solacid. They are given as 2-4 tsf two to four times in a day.

Q94. What are the drugs and dosage of H2 receptor Antagonists?

Histamine leads to secretion of Hydrochloric Acid by stimulation of H2 receptors present in the stomach wall. H2 receptor blockers compete with histamine and reduce the acid production. Four groups of H2 receptor antagonists or blockers are available – these are Cimetidine (dose 200mg twice a day), Famotidine (dose 10-20mg twice a day), Rantidine (dose 150mg twice a day) and Roxatidine (Dose 75mg twice a day). They help in the healing of ulcers in 90% cases. The commercial preparations are:

Cimetidine: Cimetidine, Tymidin, Ulciban

Ranitidine: Aciloc, Histac, Ranicure, Ranitidine,Ranitine, Rantac, Zinetac

Famotidine: Famtac, Acipep, Topcid, Famocid

Roxatidine: Rotane, Zorpex

Q95. What are the drugs and dosage of Proton Pump Inhibitors?

These groups of drugs acts on the final steps of acid production by inhibiting Proton pump or hydrogen potacium ATPase enzyme. The drugs in this group are Omeprazole (dose 20mg twice a day), Lansoprazole (dose 30mg twice a day), Pantoprazole (20-40mg once or twice a day), Rabeprazole (20mg twice a day), Esomeprazole (dose 20mg twice a day). The commercial preparations available are as follows:

Omeprazole: Omez, Oprazole, Acicure, Om, Nucid

Lansoprazole: Lan, Lancus, Lansol, Lona

Pantoprazole: Pan, Pancop 40, Pantocid, Pantodac,Pfd

Rabeprazole: Happi, Mosarab, Nucid, Cyra, Rabegon

Esomeprazole: Espra, Esoz, Sompraz

Q96. What are the drugs and dosage of Metoclopramides?

Metoclopramides increase the movement of the food in the stomach by stimulating cholinergic nerves. They also help to stop vomiting. The dosage is 5mg once or twice a day. Some of the preparations of the drug are Perinorm, Reglan, Periglo.

Q97. What are the combination therapies?

A combination of the above drugs are also used to treat peptic ulcer more effectively. The most potent drug combination is Proton Pump Inhibitor twice a day plus H2 receptor blocker at bed time. The next most effective dose is Proton Pump Inhibitor twice a day. When Lansoprozole is combined with Amoxicillin and Tinidazole (Lansikit) it can help to treat H Pylori infection in the stomach. This also helps to heal the ulcers.

Q98. What should be maintenance drugs or dosage for long-term relief after the initial treatment has given results?

After initial treatment with the most potent of them – Pantaprazole group – the ulcers can again come back in 75-90% cases after the drugs are stopped. Famotidine is less effective in healing the ulcers as compared to Pantaprazoles. But low dose – once a day ranitidine can be continued for a long time to prevent recurrence. Omeprazole 20mg once a day is also very effective for long-term maintenance treatment.

Q99. What may be the Surgical treatment of GERD?

Because GERD is often caused by a "mechanical" problem of a weakened valve of hiatal hernia, medications or lifestyle changes may not always work. For these patients, a surgical procedure could bring needed relief.

> Bile pigment is responsible in part for the yellow colour of urine. In the intestine, bilirubin is attacked by bacteria permanently stationed there and converted to a chemical known as uribilinogen which is carried to the kidneys and released in the urine.

Fundoplication involves wrapping part of the stomach around the lower esophagus, and strengthening the muscular valve. It improves the natural barrier between the stomach and the esophagus. If a hiatal hernia exists, it can be repaired at the same time.

The Nissen fundoplication can be performed by a technique called videoscopic surgery. Small tubes called trocars are inserted through 4 to 5 small incesions to create a passageway for special surgical instruments and a laparoscope. The laparoscope is a fiberoptic camera that allows the surgeon to view the organs under magnification on a video screen.

In some instances, it may be necessary for the surgeon to convert to an "open" or traditional surgery that involves a large incision, cutting across sensitive muscle tissue.

Management:

What are to be done by

Patient	Doctors	Practice
Maintain upright posture during and after eating. Stop smoking. Lose weight if you are overweight. Elevate the head of your bed 4-6 inches by placing a brick under the headboard.		✓ Avoid eating within 3 hours before bedtime. ✓ Chew non mint gum which will increase saliva production and decrease acid in the esophagus. ✓ Decrease total fat intake. ✓ Avoid stimulants.

Chapter - 5

Gastritis

Q. 100 What Is Gastritis?

Gastritis is an inflammation of the stomach. Inflammation of the stomach means the white blood cells move into the wall of the stomach as a response to an injury to the stomach. The problem is seen in two forms:

a. Acute gastritis
b. Chronic gastritis

Q 101. What is Acute Gastritis?

It is a sudden inflammation of the lining of the stomach. It occurs mainly due to overeating, overuse of alcohol, tobacco, chronic or excessive dose of aspirin, anti- inflammatory drugs, increased production of bile acids, trauma, surgery, shock, fever, jaundice, renal failure, burns, radiation therapy etc.

A germ called Helicobacter Pylori can infect the gastric mucosa and cause acute gastritis.

- Faulty dietary habits like overeating and taking highly seasoned foods.
- Bacterial toxins (salmonella, staphylococcus), metabolic toxins (uremia) and helicobacter pylori infection.

- Excessive use of alcohol, drugs (aspirin, anti-inflammatory).
- Exposure of gastric mucosa to irradiation.
- Increased production of bile salts.
- Burns and renal failure.

Q102. What are the symptoms of Acute Gastritis?

Anorexia, epigastric (upper and middle pain in the abdomen), discomfort, heartburn, nausea, severe vomiting, headache, hemorrhage and pain in the upper abdomen, dark stools, hiccups, tachycardia, rapid pulse and low blood pressure. The complications involve severe blood loss, with blood suddenly flowing into the region known as hyperemia, inflammation and even exudation.

> The gall bladder is a pear shaped, 7.5 to 12.5 cm long, with a capacity of about 50 ml, but capable of 50 fold distention. The gall bladder can store upto 0.41 litres (1/4 pints) of bile. This is emptied into the intestine through an opening in the side of the duodenum.

Q 103. What is Chronic Gastritis?

When gastritis subsides little but persists for a long duration it is called Chronic gastritis. It precedes development of organic gastric lesion, or tissue damage. Recurrent inflammation leads to changes in enzyme activity of gastric mucosal cells. Complete atrophy results in lack of absorbtion of vitamin B12 (Perinicious anaemia).

Gastroscopic observation shows 3 types of chronic gastritis:

1. **Superficial gastritis:** gastric mucous is red, oedematous, covered with adherent mucous, mucous haemorrhage and small erosion is frequently seen.
2. **Atrophic gastritis:** the mucous lining becomes thinner, gray or grayish green haemorrhage mucosa irregularly distributed.

3. **Hypertrophic gastritis:** presents a dull spongy nodular appearance of the mucosa, the edges are irregular thickened with nodular haemorrhages or superficial haemorrhages.

Q 104. What are the symptoms of Chronic Gastritis?

These include anorexia, chronic fatigue, and feeling of fullness, belching, vague epigastric pain (upper and middle pain in the abdomen), nausea and vomiting and passage of black tarry stools.

Q 105. What is the cause of Chronic Gastritis?

They are same as acute. Generally acute gastritis if well treated gets healed in 3-4 days, however if untreated can progress to chronic gastritis.

Q 106. What are the ways to diagnose Chronic Gastritis?

Confirmation of Gastritis can be done by Endoscopy. There will be a inflammation of the gastric mucosal layer. This test is much better than barium meal studies. A biopsy can also be done to know the cause of the Gastritis.

Q 107. How to confirm the cause of the Gastritis ?

The main cause of the gastritis besides food and irritant is infection of the mucosa by the bacteria helicobacter Pylori. The following special tests can be done to confirm involvement of this germ in Gastritis.

a. Elisa test for H pylori antibodies is a very appropriate test for finding this infection. This test can be also done after a successful treatment of gastritis with drugs.
b. Urea breath test: This germ H pylori releases urea gas and this can be detected by this breath test confirming the presence of this bacteria in the stomach.
c. Stool test of Antigen of H pylori can be also confirmatory.
d. Biopsy of the gastric mucosa by endoscopy can also confirm the cause being infection of H pylori.

Q.108. How to prevent Gastritis?

The best way to prevent developing gastritis is to avoid long-term use of irritants, such as aspirin, anti- inflammatory drugs and alcohol.

Q 109. What is the treatment of Gastritis?

Treatment for gastritis depends from person to person and on the specific cause. For most types of gastritis, reduction of stomach acid is helpful. Stomach acid is reduced by medication, antacids. Diet modification also controls gastritis. Antibiotics are used for infection.

Q 110. What is the diet related management of Gastritis?

Prompt medical care is successful in the management of an acute attack of gastritis only if it is accompanied by efficient and judicious nutritional care. During an acute attack of gastritis meeting the requirements is not of prime importance. Depending on the seriousness of the patient the food may be withheld for 24-48 hours. Fluid may be given intravenously if needed. Liquid foods are given as per patient's tolerance level. The amount of food and number of feedings are adjusted according to the patients tolerance, until a full regular diet is achieved. Always follow a progressive diet i.e, liquid to semi solid to solid as when the symptoms improves. The diet should contain less fat and must be bland. Many nutritional deficiencies occur in this disorder especially during chronic gastritis e.g vitamin B12, iron, and other vitamin deficiencies.

The nutritional treatment must follow general principles of soft diet. The diet should be adequate in calories and nutrients. There must be small feedings at regular intervals. Avoid gastric irritants and highly seasoned foods (onion, garlic, chilli, caffeine, cola and alcohol). Excess water or other liquids with meals may cause distention.

The dietary guidelines are enumerated here with:

Energy: give adequate calories through frequent feedings or else proteins would be utilized for energy of repair work.

Proteins: give adequate protein (1g\kg body weight) through skimmed milk, egg, steamed fish, chicken, minced meat etc.

Carbohydrates: simple easy to digest carbohydrates should be included in soft well-cooked form. Thus, semolina, rice, maida, sago, arrowroot etc. may be included whereas whole cereals and millets should particularly be avoided if gastritis has caused damage to the mucosa.

Fiber: eating a diet high in fiber reduces the risk of developing the ulcers and also speeds up healing process. However, care must be taken that fiber rich foods (soluble fiber) are always included in a soft cooked form. Raw foods seeds etc. should be completely avoided in the diet. While soluble fiber is safer for the patient as compared to insoluble fiber (husk/bran of cereals and pulses, peels of fruits and vegetables).

> The bile duct is formed by the union of common hepatic and cystic ducts. It passes downwards in front of the opening of the lesser sac between the layers of the lesser omentum, with portal vein behind and the hepatic artery on the left.

Vitamin B12: supplementation with vitamin B12 helps to treat pernicious anaemia and H. pylori infection. Its sources include fish, dairy products, organ meats, eggs, beef and pork.

Vitamin A: a combination of vitamin A (found in many green and orange coloured fruits and vegetables) and antacids is helpful in healing ulcers.

Vitamin C: a high dose of vitamin C treatment is effective in treating H. pylori infection.

It has been observe that diets high in soluble fiber, carotenoids and antioxidants reduce the risk of developing gastritis.

Food / Substances to be avoided:

Coffee with and without caffeine	Alcohol
Tobacco/ smoking	Carbonated beverages
Fruit juices with citric acid	High fat foods
Mint and vinegar	Milk
Spices	Pepper, onion and garlic

Q 111. Can Yoga help in Gastritis ?

Some of the asanas that can be practiced if suffering from gastritis are as follows:

- **Pranayama** - It is the science of breath control and consist a series of exercises intended to keep the body healthy. These exercises are to bring more oxygen to the blood and to the brain, and to control 'prana' or the vital life energy.
- **Uttanpada asana** - This asana is perfect for the people suffering from gastritis. This posture tones up the abdominal muscles and is considered as a brilliant pose for indigestion, disorders of pancreas, cures constipation and intestinal problems. This also reduces fat and wing formation in the stomach.
- **Pawanmuktasana** - The basic benefit of this asana is

to release the obstructed wing in the stomach. However, it also reduces the fat around the abdomen, strengthens the digestive system, lower back muscles, eases up the spinal vertebrae and massages the pelvic muscles and reproductive organs.

- **Bhujangasana** - This asana strengthens the spine, stretches the chest, shoulders, and abdomen, firms the buttocks, and relieves stress and fatigue.
- **Shalabhasana** - This asana is very effective in curing gastritis and improving digestion. It also strengthens the muscles of the lower back, increases flexibility in the back. It is especially recommended for relieving sciatica and pain in the lower back.
- **Vajrasana** - Other than relieving the gas from the stomach, this asana strengthens thigh muscles and calf muscles.

Practicing Yoga asana regularly reduces the occurrence of gastritis, but the person concerned should also bring changes to his diet and lifestyle. For curing gastritis, the foremost requirement is to control the diet. Healthy, balanced diet with ample of fruits and vegetables is recommended. A strict prohibition should be drawn on the consumption of spicy food, cold drinks, alcohol, street food and stale food. One should never keep the stomach empty that will invariably increase the trauma of gastritis. Short and repeated meals are the best options to keep the stomach always satiated. Smoking should be completely abolished by the person suffering from gastritis.

Q 112. What is the drug treatment of Gastritis?

The treatment of Acute or Chronic gastritis by drugs will as follows:

a. Relief of the pain in the abdomen: for this the doctor can use antispasmotic drugs like spasmindon, cyclopean or buscopan.

b. Antacids in liquid or tablet form can be used.

c. If vomiting is present – tablets like metoclopromides can be used.

d. Anti acid producing drugs like H2 receptor antagonists/ proton pump inhibitors can be used with relief.

e. To kill the H pylori bacteria four types of drugs are used in combination. These include one antibiotic(Tetracycline or Amoxycillin), anti amoebic drug like metronidazole, Proton pump inhibitors like pantaprazole and Bismuth salts (Denol, Trymo) can be used to treat H pylori for a period of 14 days. This may lead to dramatic improvement of gastritis.

Patient	Doctors	Practice
Avoid long-term use of irritants (aspirin, anti-inflammatory drugs). Stop smoking and alcohol.		✓ Take small intervals of meals ✓ Do not overeat ✓ Avoid gastric irritant and highly seasoned foods

Chapter - 6

Indigestion

Q113. What is Indigestion?

Indigestion is the term given to a group of gastrointestinal symptoms associated with the taking of food eg. nausea, heart burn, epigastric pain (upper and middle pain in the abdomen), discomfort and distension. Indigestion is not a disease, it is just a combination of complaints related to the gastro intestinal system.

Q 114. Is Indigestion and Dyspepsia same condition or different?

There is a little overlapping between the two terms. Dyspepsia is a feeling of upper abdominal pain – the major causes being peptic ulcer, GERD and gastritis. In Indigestion the abdominal pain is accompanied by discomfort, distension or nausea, loss of appetite etc. The major cause of indigestion is not a disease in the stomach but it may be just psychological disease or food intolerance. Many people consider both as same.

Q 115. What are the broad types of Indigestion?

1. Functional – This is called Irritable Bowel syndrome
2. Organic – This is due to some disease of the Gut.

In functional there is no structural change in any part of the alimentary canal. The symptoms may be psychological and emotional in origin or due to intolerance of a particular food or faulty food habits. A disease or a disorder of the digestive tract or any chronic disease of the kidney or even of the heart generally causes the second type of indigestion (organic).

Q116. What are the complaints of Indigestion problem?

> Pancreas consists of an enlarged head to the right in the concavity of the duodenum, a narrow part, the neck a body which extends to the left ending in a tail which reaches hilum of spleen. It is situated in epigastric and left hypochondriac regions and is directed nearly horizontally across posterior wall of abdomen.

The symptoms are heartburn, upper abdominal discomfort (often food related indigestion), bloating, fullness, nausea and anorexia. Such symptoms can also be seen in gatroesophageal reflux, peptic ulcer and cancer in stomach, pancrease and gallstones disease. With other organs associated, many other symptoms can be noted besides a stomach upset. These are bloating (fullness of stomach), burping, epigastric pain (upper and middle pain in the abdomen), gastrointestinal bleeding etc.

Q117. What is the cause of Indigestion?

The main etiological factor of dyspepsia is the failure of proper digestion and absorption of food in the alimentary tract and the consequences there of. Eating wrong food combinations, eating too rapidly and neglecting proper mastication and salivation of food, overeating or frequent eating produces a feverish state in the system and overtaxes the digestive organs. It produces excessive acid and causes the gastric mucous membrane to become congested. Hyperacidity is the common result. Over-eating makes the work of the stomach, liver, kidneys and bowels harder. When this food putrefies, its poisons are absorbed back into the blood and consequently, the whole system is poisoned.

Many persons, who gulp their food to stress and hurry, suffer from this ailment. When food is swallowed in large chunks, the stomach has to work harder and more hydrochloric acid is secreted. Eating too fast also causes one to swallow air. These bad habits force some of the digestive fluid into the oesophagus, causing burning, a stinging sensation or a sour taste, giving an illusion of stomach acid.

Certain foods, especially if they are not properly cooked, cause indigestion. Some people react unfavourably to certain foods like beans, cabbage, onions, cucumber, radishes and sea-foods. Fried foods as well as rich and spicy foods often cause abdominal discomfort and gas or aggravate the existing condition. Excessive smoking and intake of alcohol can also cause stomach upset. Constipation may interfere with the normal flow through the gastrointestinal tract, resulting in gas and abdominal pain. The habit of eating and drinking together is another cause of indigestion as taking liquids with meals dilutes the digestive juices and diminishes their potency. Insomnia, emotions such as jealousy, fear and anger and lack of exercise are among the other causes of this ailment.

> The peritoneum is the serous membrane of the abdominal cavity. It consists of a pariental layer lining the abdominal and pelvic walls, and a visceral layer reflected more or less over the contained organs.

Often upper abdominal pain is caused by stomach ulcer or acid reflux disease. If an individual has acid reflux disease, stomach acid backs up into the esophagus. This causes pain in the chest. Some medicine like anti-inflammatory medicines can cause indigestion. Rarely dyspepsia is caused by stomach cancer, so you should take this problem seriously. Sometimes no cause of indigestion can be found.

Q118. One of the major causes of Indigestion is Irritable Bowel Syndrome. What is this disease in actual?

Irritable Bowel Syndrome(IBS) is stress related gastrointestinal disorder which has a chronic or recurrent abdominal pain with disturbed motion (sometimes diarrhea and sometimes constipation) and often bloating. This is a very common psychological disorder where the gut seems to little sensitive and affects 10-20% of population. Medically it can be called Functional Bowel Syndrome – as it has no pathological basis.

Q119 . What are the complications of Indigestion?

Some common complications of dyspepsia/indigestion are listed below:

- Weight loss: Since eating most often provokes the symptoms, patients restrict their food. Restriction of food and skipping of meals often causes weight loss. Specific foods are also associated with symptoms e.g. fats, vegetables, milk, restriction which can result in calcium and energy deficiency.
- Altered social life: Most commonly, functional diseases interfere with the patients comfort and daily activities leading to alteration in social life.

Q. 120. What are the medical tests in case of Indigestion problem?

Indigestion is diagnosed mainly based on the symptoms. If the discomfort becomes worse or more worrisome symptoms develop (eg, severe abdominal pain, persistent nausea or vomiting or unexpected weight loss) your doctor may order one or more of the following tests:

1. Laboratory blood work
2. Barium x-ray: a chalky solution is used to highlight the upper digestive tract in x-ray
3. Ultrasound: high frequency sound waves are used to view and examine the organs of the abdominal cavity
4. Endoscopy: a long thin tube affixed with a light and camera is inserted into the throat to examine the lining of the esophagus, stomach and upper part of the small intestine
5. Gastric emptying study: food containing a small amount of radioactive material is tracked to help determine the rate at which stomach empties of food

Q121. What are the general dietary management of Indigestion?

Keeping in mind the etiology, symptoms and complications of dyspepsia it must be clear that treatment and management of this disorder does not require any major changes in the nutrient intake. All we need to take care is avoidance of a high fat diet. Modifications in the meal pattern and elimination of certain foods may however prove to be beneficial in most of the cases.

Usually bland diets are prescribed in such conditions. For excessive belching reduce the food that are gaseous (whole pulses like rajmah, channa). Soaking / sprouting whole pulses may help in making the fiber softer and hence reduce the symptoms of belching. Vegetables like radish, turnip, cauliflower, broccoli, beans and peas should be avoided.

Intolerance to lactose (the sugar in milk) often is blamed for dyspepsia. Since dyspepsia and lactose intolerance both are common, the two conditions may coexist. In this situation, restricting lactose will improve the symptoms of lactose intolerance and will also not affect the symptoms of dyspepsia.

If lactose is determined to be responsible for some or all of the symptoms, elimination of lactose containing foods is appropriate.

Lifestyle modifications:

For all types of Indigestion, it is recommended to adapt the following lifestyle changes:

- Make sure you eat regular meals.
- Lose weight if you are obese.
- If you are a smoker, consider giving up.
- Don't drink too much alcohol.

Indigestion or pain in abdomen is likely to be due to acid reflux - when heartburn is a major symptom - the following may also be worth considering:

- **Posture**. Lying down or bending forward a lot during the day encourages reflux. Sitting hunched or wearing tight belts may put extra pressure on the stomach, which may make any reflux worse.
- **Bedtime**. If symptoms recur most nights, the following may help:
  - Go to bed with an empty, dry stomach. To do this, don't eat in the last three hours before bedtime, and don't drink in the last two hours before bedtime.
  - If you are able, try raising the head of the bed by 10-20 cms (for example, with books or bricks under the bed's legs). This helps gravity to keep acid from refluxing into the oesophagus. If you do this, do not use additional pillows, because this may increase abdominal pressure.

Q122. What are the yogasanas for Indigestion?

ARDHA MATSYENDRASANA

It is highly recommended for treatment of obesity, dyspepsia, diabetes and urinary disorders. One should not do this asana forcibly.

Steps

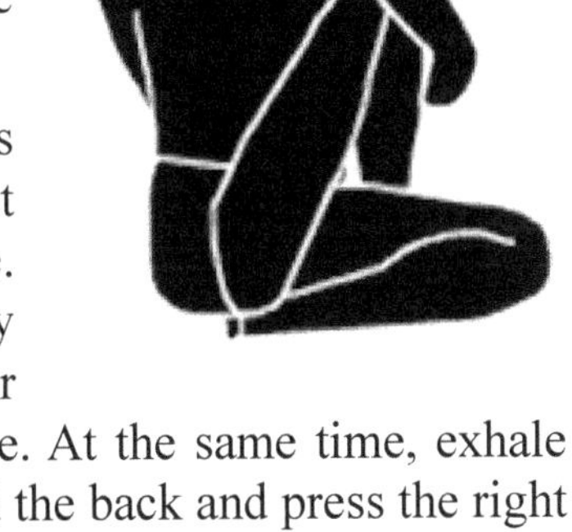

- Sit on the ground, stretching both the legs forward. Bend your right leg and place the heel under the left hip.
- Now bend your left leg, cross it over and place your foot by the side of the right knee. Try to hold the left ankle by passing the right arm over the left side of the left knee. At the same time, exhale and take the left arm behind the back and press the right side under the ribs.
- This has to be done by twisting the trunk to the back as much as possible. Maintain this posture for a few seconds and increase the duration to two minutes gradually.
- Repeat the same process on the other side for the same duration.

SHIRSHASANA

Shirshaasana is also called the king of the yoga poses. The practice in which the navel is above and the palate below, the Sun above and the Moon below is known as Viparitakarani (topsy turvy pose), it can be learnt from the words uttered by a Guru. On the first day, one should remain for a very short time with one's head below and feet above. The duration of this practice should be gradually increased day by day.

Steps

- Sit on soles. Place knees on the ground.
- Frame finger lock with both hands.
- Making a triangle from finger-lock and elbows, place it on ground.
- Now straighten your legs.
- Slowly bring the legs near your body.
- Soles will automatically leave the ground by practice and thighs and knees will touch the abdomen.
- Now keeping the balance straighten your legs from thigh-joint, knees will remain folded.
- Now straighten the knees also and completely balance your body on head.
- While returning to the original position fold your knee first. Then fold your legs from thigh and let the thigh and knee touch your abdomen.
- Now slowly place the soles on the ground. Slowly raise your head also and sit on soles.

SARVANGA ASANA

The Sarvanga Asana is one of the most treasured asanas, said to benefit the whole body. In this asana, the whole body weight rests on the shoulders and the neck and upper ba stretched to the limit. Beginners should practic asana in a moderate way and gradually attempt tl

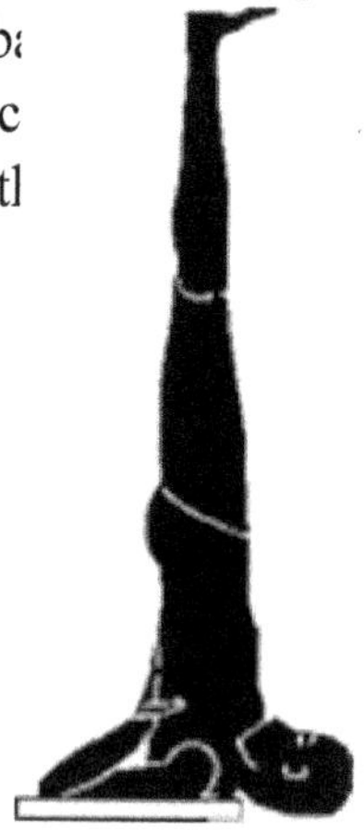

Steps

- Lie straight, on your back on the floor. Palms should be on the floor close to the body and the heels and the toes should be together.
- Inhale and raise both the legs slowly up in a vertical position (at 90o). Raising

of the legs should be synchronized with the breathing.

- Exhale and again raise the legs upward from the second position. Bring both palms underneath the hips and should be used to assist in raising the body upwards. The hands should always work as a support to the body weight.
- Try to raise the body as straight as possible.
- At the final stage of this asana you will be resting on your shoulders, chin touching the chest. In this position the legs should be stiff hard and together and the toes is pointing towards the ceiling. Do not shake. Be firm and keep breathing normally.
- Remain in this position for about 30 seconds on the first day.
- For returning to the first position, first fold the legs on the knees. Your heels should be now on the thighs and above the buttock. Then slowly let the body return to the floor while the palms are supporting the body weight.
- Now stretch out the legs forwards and relax. You have completed one round of the Sarvanga Asana.

Chapter - 7

Irritable Bowel Syndrome or Stress related Disease of Gut

Q123. How many people are affected by this disease called IBS (Irritable Bowel Syndrome)?

With the increasing stress in life, the number of people suffering from IBS all over the world especially in the developing country. It is said that 50% of the diarrhoea patients in a Government hospital OPD are suffering from IBS. This is also called stress related loose motion. This disease is more common in the lower economic class and in young people. More ladies are affected compared to the gents. This disease decreases with age.

Q124. What are the symptoms of Irritable Bowel Syndrome ?

Pain in the abdomen, bowel disturbance in the form of constipation or diarrhoea, urgency of passing stool, feeling of incomplete evacuation or

> The appendix is a narrow shaped piece of the intestine hanging from the caecum. It has no apparent use in the body. The appendix varies in length and circumference. The average length is between 7.5 and 10 cm. The appendix averages 05 cm longer in male than in the female.

passing of mucous are some of the typical symptoms of IBS. Most of these symptoms occur for a small period and not present continuously for days or weeks. Many a times distension of the abdomen is also associated with IBS. The pain in the abdomen is not localised and keep on varying in nature and migrate in the abdomen. This pain is not relieved by passing of the stool, mostly not related to any activity, urination or menstruation.

Many patients of IBS present with infrequent defecation, straining with defecation or incomplete evacuation.

The symptoms of GERD(heart burn) may be present in 30% of IBS patients. Some complain of headache, backache, fatigue.

Q125. What are the diseases that the IBS is confused with?

These are:

a. Constipation
b. Diarrhoea
c. Inflammatory bowel disease
d. Colitis
e. Depression
f. Intestinal infections
g. Cancer

Q126. What are the symptoms that go against IBS or stress induced Bowel disease?

The following symptoms go against the diagnosis of IBS:

a. Weight loss
b. Dysphagia (problems in swallowing)
c. Evidence of dehydration or bleeding
d. Recurrent vomiting

e. Fever

f. Fatty stool

Q127. How to confirm the diagnosis of IBS?

When we exclude the presence of all the other possible diseases – the diagnosis point towards IBS. Most of the patients show symptoms of anxity, depression and excessive stress.

The following tests can be done to exclude other diseases:

a. Blood count, Hb, ESR	to exclude Anaemia, inflammation
b. Lever function test, electrolytes	to exclude liver disease, electrolyte disturbance
c.Thyroid hormones	to exclude thyroid diseases
d. Stool for blood	to exclude bleeding
e. Rectal endoscopy	to exclude colitis, cancer
f. Stool	to exclude diarrhoea, germs
g. Lactose tolerance test	to exclude lactose intolerance

Q128. How stress leads to all the symptoms like pain in the abdomen, diarrhoea, constipation or distension of the abdomen or feeling of incomplete passage of stool?

Abdominal pain is due to sensitive colon. The colon responds vigorously to meals, there is contraction of colon muscles which become sensitive.

Constipation occurs due to absence of high-grade peristalsis which push the stool, reduced emptying of ascending and transverse colon.

Diarrhoea occurs due to increased colonic contractions, increased fluid secretion of fluid in response to bile acids, increased colon actions during fasting period.

Bloating or distension occurs due to intestinal hypersensitivity, less expulsion of gas. Rectum also becomes hyper sensitive which leads to the feeling of incomplete evacuation.

Q129. What is the line of treatment for IBS?

The line of treatment:

a. Reassurance
b. Diet
c. Meditation and Yoga
d. Stress management
e. Medicines

Q130. What are the ways to reassure the patients of IBS?

The patient must be told that problem is real and they are very common in general population. The assurance should also tell the patient that there is no life-threatening situation possible out of this problem – like cancer. Providing an early correct diagnosis, spending time to explain the possible causes of the symptoms, telling them to be less concerned and take symptomatic treatment is good enough for the patients. Many of them do not need any treatment once they are assured.

> The anus or the anal canal is about 10 cm (4 inch) long and is the opening through which the body's solid waste products - known as faeces are excreated. The caecum is a blind pouch from which the large intestine starts. The ileum, the last of the divisions of the small intestines, opens into the caecum. The appendix projects from it.

Q131. What are the dietary management of IBS?

Patients of IBS should be prescribed a high fiber diet – almost double than what they usually take. Some high fiber diet may cause gas formation ; in such cases isabgol or other fibre preparations can be given – gradually increasing the dosage from one dose to two weekly – till the symptoms improve.

Cabbage, beans, lentils should be avoided by the patients as they produce a lot of gas and flatulence.

Q132. What are the Stress management techniques that can improve the patients?

a. Yoga/ mediatation

b. Phycho therapy

c. Development of positive attitude

d. Changing of mindset and understanding of reality

e. Regular walk, exercise

Q 133. What are the drugs for treating IBS?

Because the symptoms of IBS are related to stress/ psychology and not because of any disease, the drug treatment is not so satisfactory. Often just a vitamin pill can give relief to 30-70% patents – even if the patient knows that he /she is taking just a vitamin pill. This is also partly because the patient also do not have these symptoms always and intermittent relief is also taken as if the pill has worked.

Only when the symptoms reach a severe stage, patients usually report to the physician and have mostly spontaneous improvement. So, the drugs should be avoided in such patients and only relief of the symptoms should be tried. The patients should be asked what is the main difficulty – abdominal pain or diarrhoea or constipation or just distension and accordingly the symptoms must be treated. Often the patients go back after reassurance and mostly discontinue the drugs after a short while on their own.

The diaphragm is a sheet of muscle which forms a barrier between the contents of the chest and those of the abdomen.

If the symptoms really become more antidepression/mood elevator medicines, sleeping pills can be prescribed.

Q134. What are the medicines prescribed to such patients of Irritable Bowel Symdrome?

For Constipation: Bulk purgatives like Cremalax, Isobgol, Cremaffin; Osmotic purgatives like Milk of magnesium, Lactulose; enemas can be given.

For Diarrhoea : Lopramide (Lomotil, Lomofen, Lopramide), Simethicon can be given.

For Abdominal pain: Anti spasmodic drugs like baralgan, cyclopean, spamindon can be given.

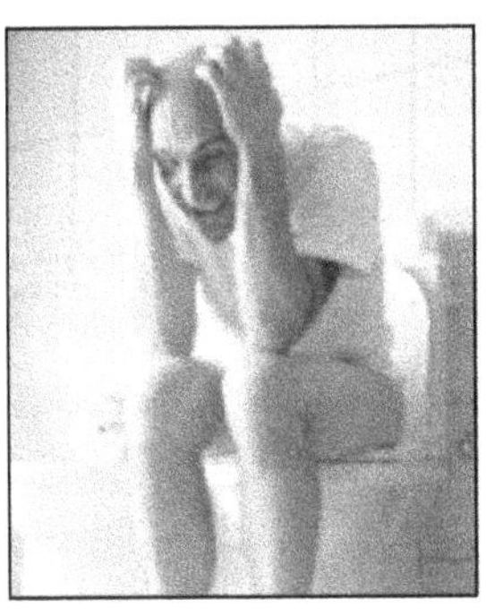

For Flatulence or Gas: Enzyme preparations like Aristozyme, Fastal N, Gaskit, Pancreaflat can be given.

For Depression: Amitryptiline, Doxpin, Imipramine, Nortryptiline, Trazodone, Floxetine can be given.

Chapter - 8

Constipation & Piles

Q 135. What is Constipation?

Constipation is irregular, infrequent or difficulty in passage of faeces. It is the most common disorder of the alimentary tract. It is characterized by evacuation of hard, dried stools. It occurs commonly in children, adolescents and adults age 65 and over who take low fiber diets and patients confined to bed. It is a condition in which fewer than 3 stools per week are passed. If more than 3 days go by - without the passage of a stool and stool passed in one day amounting to less than 35 grams, it can be called Constipation.

People who are constipated may find it difficult and painful to have a bowel movement. Other symptoms of constipation include feeling bloated, uncomfortable and sluggish.

> The fat provides a good source of energy as glucose, but in doing so it produces extra waste products called ketones.

Many people think they are constipated even when their bowel movements are regular. For example, some people believe they are constipated, or irregular if they do not have a bowel movement every day. However, there is no right number of daily or weekly bowel movements. Normal may be three times a day or three times a week depending on the person. Also, some people naturally have firmer stools than others. At one time or the other, everyone gets constipated. Poor diet and lack of exercise are usually the causes. In most cases, constipation is temporary and not serious. Understanding its causes, prevention and treatment will help most people find relief.

Q136. What are the types of Constipation?

There are three main types of constipation. These are:

a. Atonic Constipation
b. Spastic Constipation
c. Obstructive Constipation

Ketones do not appear in the blood until several hours after a balanced meal. By the time most of us wake up in the morning, we are slightly ketotic: small amounts of ketones are present in the blood and urine. Much of the energy for an early morning jog would be supplied to the muscles by these ketones, which disappear from the bloodstream after a good breakfast.

Q137. What is Atonic type of Constipation?

It is the most common type of constipation. During the process of digestion the food particles (half digested or after digestion is over) are moved in the gut by a movement called Peristalsis. This is a rhythmic movement of the intestinal wall which propels the food towards the rectum and ultimately leading the leftover food out through the anus. In Atonic type of constipation, the intestinal walls lack muscular tone so that peristaltic action is impaired. The food mass thus cannot move at a normal rate down the tract. Bacterial action may be greatly increased owing to the stagnation of material in the colon and possibly the products of this action may be responsible for at least some of the symptoms usually occurring as a result of constipation. The chief causes of atonic constipation are selection of foods low in bulk, insufficient fluids, poor personal hygiene, lack of exercise, chronic illness, pregnancy or excessive use of enemas.

Q138. What is Spastic type of Constipation?

This is characterized by increased tonicity of the musculature. The contractions throughout the tract act in a spasmodic manner, causing the movement of the food mass to be very irregular. Spasmodic movements cause acute pain.

Spastic constipation may be caused by irritation of the intestinal mucosa through the excessive use of alcohol, spices, tea, coffee, bran or laxatives. Highly strung, nervous people are more frequently affected by this type of constipation.

> When glucose is scarce, fatty tissues is broken down into fatty acids and carried in the bloodstream to the liver, where ketone bodies are formed.

Q139. What is an Obstructive type of Constipation?

It occurs usually due to obstruction in the colon or any other obstruction due to inflammation or narrowing of the lumen. Hard stool getting impacted in the rectum is one of the main reasons of this type of constipation.

Q140. What are the main causes of temporary Constipation?

Temporary constipation can be due to any one of a number of factors such as:

- Inadequate diet
- Failure to establish regular times for eating, adequate rest, and elimination
- Faulty dietary habits, such as inadequate fluid and fiber

intake or use of highly refined and concentrated foods that leaves little residue in the colon

- Interference with the urge to defecate brought on by illness, nervous tension, or a trip away from home
- Changes in one's usual routine brought on by illness, nervous tension, or a trip away from home
- Chronic use of laxatives
- Difficult or painful defecation due to hemorrhoids or fissures
- Poor muscle tone of the intestine and stasis due to lack of exercise occurring especially in bed ridden patients, invalids such as arthritics, the aged and others
- Organic disorders such as diverticulosis or obstruction from adhesions or neoplasms
- Ingestion of drugs, large amounts of sedatives, ganglionic blocking agents or opiates
- Spasm of intestine due to presence of irritating material, psychogenic influences or others

Q141. What are the causes of Constipation?

> Faeces are usually composed of about 75% water and 25% solid material. Some of the water is mucus which lubricates the alimentary canal and eases the passage of faeces from the body.

To understand constipation, it helps to know how the colon, or large intestine, works. As food moves through the colon, the colon absorbs water from the food while it forms waste products, or stool. Muscle contractions in the colon then push the stool toward the rectum. By the time stool reaches the rectum it is solid, because most of the water has been absorbed.

Constipation occurs when the colon absorbs too much water or if the colon's muscle contractions are slow or sluggish, causing the stool to move through the colon too slowly. As a result, stools can become hard and dry. Common causes of constipation are:

- not enough fiber in the diet
- not enough liquids
- lack of physical activity (especially in the elderly)
- medications
- irritable bowel syndrome
- changes in life or routine such as pregnancy, aging, and travel
- abuse of laxatives
- ignoring the urge to have a bowel movement
- specific diseases or conditions, such as stroke (most common)
- problems with the colon and rectum
- problems with intestinal function (chronic idiopathic constipation)

Q142. Why is it common that the fiber is missing from the diet? How fiber helps to avoid Constipation?

People who eat a high-fiber diet are less likely to become constipated. The most common causes of constipation are a diet low in fiber or a diet high in fats, such as cheese, eggs, and meats.

> The colour of the faeces is due to the bile pigment (chemical break down products of red blood cells) called stercobilin and bilirubin. These bile pigments also help to sterilize and deodorize faeces.

Fiber—both soluble and insoluble—is the part of fruits, vegetables, and grains that the body cannot digest. Soluble fiber dissolves easily in water and takes on a soft, gel-like texture in the intestines. Insoluble fiber passes through the intestines almost unchanged. The bulk and soft texture of fiber help prevent hard, dry stools that are difficult to pass.

Our food is generally low in fiber. Both children and adults often eat too many refined and processed foods from which the natural fiber has been removed.

> Glucose, a simple sugar, is the main source of energy for the body's cells. It is extracted from starches and sweet foods.

A low-fiber diet also plays a key role in constipation among older adults, who may lose interest in eating and choose foods that are quick to make or buy, such as fast foods, or prepared foods, both of which are usually low in fiber. Also, difficulties with chewing or swallowing may cause older people to eat soft foods that are processed and low in fiber.

Q143.What happens when the liquids are not there in food?

Research shows that although increased fluid intake does not necessarily help relieve constipation, many people report some relief from their constipation if they drink fluids such as water and juice and avoid dehydration. Liquids add fluid to the colon and bulk to stools, making bowel movements softer and easier to pass. People who have problems with constipation should try to drink liquids every day. However, liquids that contain caffeine, such as coffee and cola drinks will worsen one's symptoms by causing dehydration. Alcohol is another beverage that causes dehydration. It is important to drink fluids that hydrate the body, especially when consuming caffeine containing drinks or alcoholic beverages.

> Glucose, a simple sugar, is the main source of energy for the body's cells. It is extracted from starches and sweet foods.

Q144. Why lack of Physical Activity lead to Constipation?

A lack of physical activity can lead to constipation, although doctors do not know precisely why. For example, constipation often occurs after an accident or during an illness when one must stay in bed and cannot exercise. Lack of physical activity is thought to be one of the reasons constipation is common in older people.

Q 145. What kind of medicines lead to Constipation?

Almost all the allopathic medicines may lead to some constipation but some of them are definitely constipative. Some medications that can cause constipation are:

- pain medications (especially narcotics)
- antacids that contain aluminum and calcium
- blood pressure medications (calcium channel blockers)
- antiparkinson drugs
- antispasmodics
- antidepressants
- iron supplements
- diuretics
- anticonvulsants

Q146. Can Constipation occur due to psychological problem like stress?

In the busy world of today, almost none can escape the effects of stress on the body. Many health condition are caused or exacerbated by stress. Constipation is not exceptional. There are two major ways in which stress can affect constipation. First, stress causes us to make lifestyle choices that are unhealthy for the intestinal tract. Secondly, stress can change the patterns of digestion.

> Glycogen, a form of glucose, is stored in the liver and muscles and released as needed for energy.

Some people with IBS (Irritable Bowel Syndrome), also known as spastic colon, have spasms in the colon that affect bowel movements. Constipation and diarrhea often alternate, and abdominal cramping, gassiness, and bloating are other common complaints. Although, IBS can produce lifelong symptoms, it is not a life-threatening condition. It often worsens with stress, but there is no specific cause or anything unusual that the doctor can see in the colon.

Q 147. Can changes in life or routine cause Constipation?

During pregnancy, women may be constipated because of hormonal changes or because the uterus compresses the intestine. Aging may also affect bowel regularity, because a slower metabolism results in less intestinal activity and muscle tone. In addition, people often become constipated when traveling, because their normal diet and daily routine are disrupted.

Q 148. Can excess use of Laxatives lead to Constipation?

The common belief that people must have a daily bowel movement has led to self-medicating with OTC (over the counter drugs) laxative products. Although people may feel relief when they use laxatives, typically they must increase the dose over time because the body grows reliant on laxatives in order to have a bowel movement. As a result, laxatives may become habit-forming.

Q149. Can ignoring the urge to have a bowel movement lead to Constipation?

People who ignore the urge to have a bowel movement may eventually stop feeling the need to have one, which can lead to constipation. Some people delay having a bowel movement because they do not want to use toilets outside the home. Others ignore the urge because of emotional stress or because they are too busy. Children may postpone having a bowel movement because of stressful toilet training or because they do not want to interrupt their play.

Q150. What are the diseases that can lead to Constipation?

Diseases that cause constipation include neurological disorders, metabolic and endocrine disorders, and systemic conditions that affect organ systems. These disorders can slow the movement of stool through the colon, rectum, or anus.

Conditions that can cause constipation are found below:

> Insulin is a hormone which is made in the pancreas and which lowers the level of sugar in the blood.

- Neurological disorders
    - multiple sclerosis
    - Parkinson's disease
    - chronic idiopathic intestinal pseudo-obstruction
    - stroke
    - spinal cord injuries
- Metabolic and endocrine conditions
    - diabetes
    - uremia
    - hypercalcemia

- poor glycemic control
- hypothyroidism

➢ Systemic disorders

- amyloidosis
- lupus
- scleroderma

Q 151. Can Constipation occur due to problems with the Colon and Rectum?

Intestinal obstruction, scar tissue—also called adhesions—diverticulosis, tumors, colorectal stricture, Hirschsprung disease, or cancer can compress, squeeze, or narrow the intestine and rectum and cause constipation.

> Diarrhoea is due to the increased number of osmotically active oligosaccharide molecules that remain in the intestinal lumen, causing the volume of the intestinal contents to increase.

Q 152. What is Functional Constipation?

The two types of constipation are idiopathic constipation and functional constipation. Irritable Bowel Syndrome (IBS) with predominant symptoms of constipation is categorized separately.

Idiopathic—of unknown origin—constipation does not respond to standard treatment.

Functional constipation means that the bowel is healthy but not working properly. Functional constipation is often the result of poor dietary habits and lifestyle. It occurs in both children and adults and is most common in women. Colonic inertia, delayed transit, and pelvic floor dysfunction are three types of functional constipation. Colonic inertia and delayed transit are caused by a decrease in muscle activity in the colon. These syndromes may affect the entire colon or may be confined to the lower, or sigmoid, colon.

> Bloating and flatulence are due to the production of gas (CO_2 and H_2) from disaccharide residues in the lower small intestine and colon.

Pelvic floor dysfunction is caused by a weakness of the muscles in the pelvis surrounding the anus and rectum. However, because this group of muscles is voluntarily controlled to some extent, biofeedback training is somewhat successful in retraining the muscles to function normally and improving the ability to have a bowel movement.

Functional constipation that stems from problems in the structure of the anus and rectum is known as anorectal dysfunction, or anismus. These abnormalities result in an inability to relax the rectal and anal muscles that allow stool to exit.

Q 153. What way we should proceed for Diagnosis of Constipation?

The tests, the doctor performs, depend on the duration and severity of the constipation, the person's age, and whether blood in stools, recent changes in bowel habits, or weight loss have occurred. Most people with constipation do not need extensive testing and can be treated with changes in diet and exercise. For example, in young people with mild symptoms, a medical history and physical exam may be all that is needed for diagnosis and treatment.

Medical History

The doctor may ask a patient to describe his or her constipation, including duration of symptoms, frequency of bowel movements, consistency of stools, presence of blood in the stool, and toilet habits—how often and where one has bowel movements. A record of eating habits, medication, and level of physical activity will also help the doctor determine the cause of constipation.

The clinical definition of constipation is having any two of the following symptoms for at least 12 weeks—not always consecutive—in the previous 12 months:

- straining during bowel movements
- lumpy or hard stool
- sensation of incomplete evacuation
- sensation of anorectal blockage/obstruction
- fewer than three bowel movements per week

Q154. What are the physical examinations that should be performed in case of Constipation?

A physical exam may include a rectal exam with a gloved, lubricated finger to evaluate the tone of the muscle that closes off the anus—also called anal sphincter—and to detect tenderness, obstruction, or blood.

Q 155. What are the medical tests for Constipation?

Extensive testing usually is reserved for people with severe symptoms, for those with sudden changes in the number and consistency of bowel movements or blood in the stool, and older adults. Additional tests that may be used to evaluate constipation include:

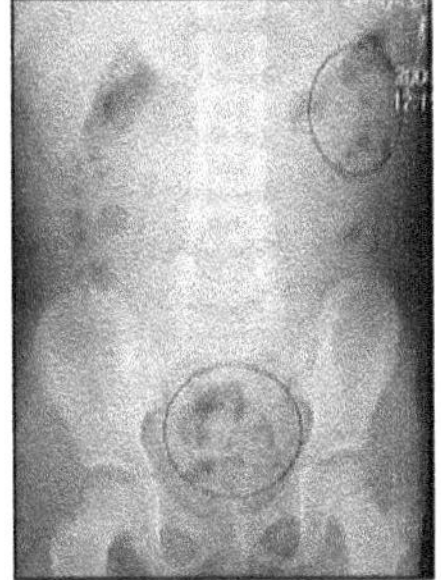

- a colorectal transit study
- anorectal function tests
- a defecography

Because of an increased risk of colorectal cancer in older adults, the doctor may use tests to rule out a diagnosis of cancer, including:

- barium enema x ray
- sigmoidoscopy or colonoscopy

In some cases, blood and thyroid tests may be necessary to look for thyroid disease and serum calcium or to rule out inflammatory, metabolic, and other disorders.

Q156. What is Colorectal transit study?

This test shows how well food moves through the colon. The patient swallows capsules containing small markers that are visible on an x ray. The movement of the markers through the colon is monitored by abdominal x rays taken several times 3 to 7 days after the capsule is swallowed. The patient eats a high-fiber diet during the course of this test.

Q 157. What are the anorectal function tests?

> The problem of milk intolerance can be relieved by administration of commercial lactase preparations. Even yoghurt can be tolerated because it contains its own bacterial lactase.

These tests diagnose constipation caused by abnormal functioning of the anus or rectum—also called anorectal function.

- **Anorectal manometry** evaluates anal sphincter muscle function. For this test, a catheter or air-filled balloon is inserted into the anus and slowly pulled back through the sphincter muscle to measure muscle tone and contractions.
- **Balloon expulsion tests** consist of filling a balloon with varying amounts of water after it has been rectally inserted. Then the patient is asked to expel the balloon. The inability to expel a balloon filled with less than 150 ml of water may indicate a decrease in bowel function.

- **Defecography** is an x ray of the anorectal area that evaluates completeness of stool elimination, identifies anorectal abnormalities, and evaluates rectal muscle contractions and relaxation. During the exam, the doctor fills the rectum with a soft paste that is the same consistency as stool. The patient sits on a toilet positioned inside an x-ray machine, then relaxes and squeezes the anus to expel the paste. The doctor studies the x rays for anorectal problems that occurred as the paste was expelled.

Q158. What is Barium enema x ray?

This exam involves viewing the rectum, colon, and lower part of the small intestine to locate problems. This part of the digestive tract is known as the bowel. This test may show intestinal obstruction and Hirschsprung disease, which is a lack of nerves within the colon.

The night before the test, bowel cleansing, also called bowel prep, is necessary to clear the lower digestive tract. The patient drinks a special liquid to flush out the bowel. A clean bowel is important, because even a small amount of stool in the colon can hide details and result in an incomplete exam.

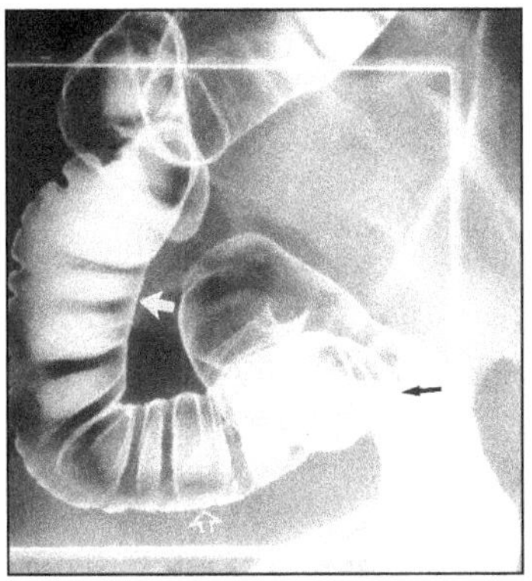

Because the colon does not show up well on x rays, the doctor fills it with barium, a chalky liquid that makes the area visible. Once the mixture coats the inside of the colon and rectum, x rays are taken that show their shape and condition. The patient may feel some abdominal cramping when the barium fills the colon but usually feels little discomfort after the procedure. Stools may be white in color for a few days after the exam.

Q159. What is Sigmoidoscopy or Colonoscopy?

An examination of the rectum and lower, or sigmoid, colon is called a sigmoidoscopy. An examination of the rectum and entire colon is called a colonoscopy.

The person usually has a liquid dinner the night before a colonoscopy or sigmoidoscopy and takes an enema early the next morning. An enema an hour before the test may also be necessary.

> In humans, a congenital defect in the mechanism that transports amino acids in the intestine and renal tubules causes Hartnup disease.

To perform a sigmoidoscopy, the doctor uses a long, flexible tube with a light on the end, called a sigmoidoscope, to view the rectum and lower colon. The patient is lightly sedated before the exam. First, the doctor examines the rectum with a gloved, lubricated finger. Then, the sigmoidoscope is inserted through the anus into the rectum and lower colon. The procedure may cause abdominal pressure and a mild sensation of wanting to move the bowels. The doctor may fill the colon with air to get a better view. The air can cause mild cramping.

To perform a colonoscopy, the doctor uses a flexible tube with a light on the end, called a colonoscope, to view the entire colon. This tube is longer than a sigmoidoscope. During the exam, the patient lies on his or her side, and the doctor inserts the tube through the anus and rectum into the colon. If an abnormality is seen, the doctor can use the colonoscope to remove a small piece of tissue for examination (biopsy). The patient may feel gassy and bloated after the procedure.

> Fatty acids containing less than 10-12 carbon atoms pass from the mucosal cells directly into the portal blood, where they are transported as free fatty acids. The fatty acids containing more than 10-12 carbon atoms are reesterified to triglycerides in the mucosal cells.

Q160. What are the lifestyle changes suggested to treat or prevent Constipation?

When we are busy and stressed, we tend not to take care of our bodies. Being busy can cause many to wait to go to the bathroom. Delaying a bowel movement is one of the most common reasons that people become constipated. A stressful schedule can also lead many people to eat on the run. Most "fast-food" diets include large portions of meat, fat, and soda and very few protions of vegetables, whole grains, and water. This type of diet can often lead to stress and constipation. People often skip meals and eat hurriedly, not taking the time to chew their food. Because a regular schedule of eating leads to regular bowel movements, irregular eating can lead to problems with stress and constipation.

If you have constipation as a result of stress, there are many options that you can choose to prevent this problem.

> The intestines are presented each day with about 2000 ml of ingested fluid plus 700 ml secreted from the mucosa of the gastrointestinal tract and associated glands.

Exercise can be a great stress reliever and has added benefit of promoting healthy digestion. It may seem like just one more thing to add to your schedule but it will be worth it. Planning meals ahead of time can help with some constipation problems. Instead of skipping meals, keep healthy snacks on hand for busy days. If you have to eat on the run choose option with healthier meals. Many fast food restaurants are offering healthy options that include vegetables. Keep water with you at all times. If you have a bottle of water on your desk or in the car, you'll be more likely to stay hydrated. If you're suffering from severe symptoms of constipation as a result of stress, it is a good idea to talk to your healthcare provider. Together you can come up with a solution to improve both your physical health and your mental health.

Q 161. What are the complications of Constipation?

Constipation, if present for a long time and not taken care can lead to two common complications. These complications include piles or hemorrhoids, caused by straining to have a bowel movement and anal fissures – tears in the skin around the anus—caused when hard stool stretches the sphincter muscle. As a result, rectal bleeding may occur, appearing as bright red streaks on the surface of the stool.

Other complications of constipation are fecal impaction and rectal prolapse.

> Food in the stomach accelerates the increase in gastric secretion produced by the sight and smell of the food and the presence of food in the mouth. Receptors in the wall of the stomach and the mucosa respond to stretch and chemical stimuli, mainly amino acids and related products of digestion.

Q162. What is Piles or Hemorrhoids and how to treat it?

When we pass hard stools they pressurise and scratch the soft mucous membrane lining the wall of the anus, the last end of the gut. This leads to bleeding from the engorged veins and many a times a reddish or purple mass also comes out of the anus. This condition is very common and termed Piles or haemorrhoids. In initial cases, there is only bleeding, but in severe cases it may have bleeding plus permanent prolapsed where a mass comes out of the anal aperture. The bright red coloured blood is usually seen as a thin line sticking all along the wall of the hard passing stool. When the bleeding is more frank blood can come in drops. Mostly there is no pain.

The treatment involves softening of the stools by use of soft laxatives for a period of two weeks so that the wound in the mucous membrane can heal. Avoiding constipation producing foods, eating high fibre food and lots of liquid also help to soften the stool. If the constipation continues, the piles start bleeding again and have more complications.

Surgery is only indicated when the medical management fails. Elastic band ligation, injections of sclerosing liquids, photo coagulation, cryo surgery and lastly excision of the affected veins are the possible surgical treatment.

Foods rich in carbohydrates leaves the stomach in few hours. Protein rich food leaves more slowly, and emptying is slowest after a meal containing fat. The rate of emptying also depends on the osmotic pressure of the material entering the duodenum.

Treatment for hemorrhoids may include warm tub baths, ice packs, and application of a special cream to the affected area.

Q163. What is Anal Fissure and how to treat it?

This is a split in the skin around the anal outlet. This fissures mostly result from a vigorous stretching of the anal canal, most commonly during defecation by a large, hard stool mass. Previous surgical procedure in the anal area leading to fibrosis of the area also makes it easy to happen. The fissures are usually accompanied by severe anal pain, especially during passing of hard stool. The pain is so much that patients often fear to pass stool and this further complicated the situation. Many a times there is bleeding from the fissure.

The medical treatment involves stool softeners, bulk purgatives, and sitz bath (lying down on a tumbler of warm water) and can lead to healing in 90% of fissures. Local anaesthetic creams, steroid creams can also be applied just before defecation to give pain relief to the patient during passage of stool. Injection of botulinum toxin can be tried which alter the nerve end in that area giving pain relief. Surgical correction is the last resort but can give good results in bad cases.

Treatment for anal fissures may include stretching the sphincter muscle or surgically removing the tissue or skin in the affected area.

Q164. What is rectal prolapsed and how to treat it?

Sometimes straining causes a small amount of intestinal lining to push out from the anal opening. This condition, known as rectal prolapse, may lead to secretion of mucus from the anus. Usually eliminating the cause of the prolapse, such as straining or coughing, is the only treatment necessary. Severe or chronic prolapse requires surgery to strengthen and tighten the anal sphincter muscle or to repair the prolapsed lining.

Q165. What is Fecal impaction and how to treat it?

> The pancreatic juice is alkaline and has high bicarbonate content. About 1500 ml of pancreatic juice is secreted per day.

Constipation may also cause hard stool to pack the intestine and rectum so tightly that the normal pushing action of the colon is not enough to expel the stool. This condition, called fecal impaction, occurs most often in children and older adults. An impaction can be softened with mineral oil taken by mouth and by an enema. After softening the impaction, the doctor may break up and remove part of the hardened stool by inserting one or two fingers into the anus.

Q 166. How is Constipation treated?

Although treatment depends on the cause, severity, and duration of the constipation, in most cases dietary and lifestyle changes will help relieve symptoms and help prevent them from recurring. Use of laxatives and enamas can be recommended once the diet and lifestyle measures fail.

Diet:

A diet with enough fiber (20 to 35 grams each day) helps the body form soft, bulky stool. A doctor or dietitian can help plan an appropriate diet. High-fiber foods include beans, whole grains and bran cereals, fresh fruits, and vegetables such as asparagus, brussels sprouts, cabbage, and carrots. For people prone to constipation, limiting foods that have little or no fiber, such as ice cream, cheese, meat, and processed foods, is also important.

Lifestyle Changes:

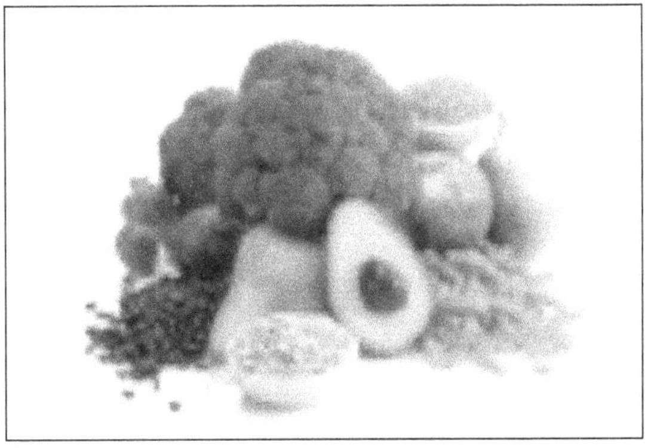

Other changes that may help treat and prevent constipation include drinking enough water and other liquids, such as fruit and vegetable juices and clear soups, so as not to become dehydrated, engaging in daily exercise, and reserving enough time to have a bowel movement. In addition, the urge to have a bowel movement should not be ignored.

Q 167. What are the Laxatives used for treatment of Constipation?

Most people who are mildly constipated do not need laxatives. However, for those who have made diet and lifestyle changes and are still constipated, a doctor may recommend laxatives or enemas for a limited time. These treatments can help retrain a chronically sluggish bowel. For children, short-term treatment with laxatives, along with retraining to establish regular bowel habits, helps prevent constipation.

People who are dependent on laxatives need to slowly stop using them. A doctor can assist in this process. For most people, stopping laxatives restores the colon's natural ability to contract.

A doctor should determine when a patient needs a laxative and which form is best. Laxatives taken by mouth are available in liquid, tablet, gum powder, and granule forms. They work in various ways.

Q168. What are the kinds of laxatives used?

The major types of laxatives can be devided according to their mode of action. They are:

a. Bulk forming Laxatives
b. Stimulant Laxatives
c. Osmotic laxatives
d. Stool softeners
e. Lubricants
f. Herbal formulations
g. Plant Mucus of the Bassorin series

Q 169. What are the Bulk forming laxatives and how do they work?

> Gallstones occurs in 10-20% of the population and in the western societies, 85% of the stones are cholesterol stones.

Bulk-forming laxatives generally are considered the safest, but they can interfere with absorption of some medicines. These laxatives, also known as fiber supplements, are taken with water. They absorb water in the intestine and make the stool softer. Some of the bulk laxatives are bran, psyllium, ispaghula, methyl cellulose . These agents must be taken with water or they can cause obstruction. Many people also report no relief after taking bulking agents and suffer from a worsening in bloating and abdominal pain if there is fermentation of these fibres in the intestine.

Some of the commercial preparations are Fibril, Feel Good, Isabgol, Fibernut, Fybrogel, Naturolax, Softovac.

Q170. What are the stimulant laxatives and how do they work?

In man, the protein turnover involves breakdown and resynthesis of 80-100 gms of tissue protein per day and about 50% part occurs in the liver.

Stimulants cause rhythmic muscle contractions in the intestines. They are also called contact purgatives. The compounds are Dipheyl-methanes, Phenolphthalein, bisacodyl, Anthraquinoles. Anthraquinoles include senna, cascara, sagrada, fixed oil, castor oil. Some of the commercially available preparations are Dulcolax, Julax, Agarol, Sofsena, Glaxena.

Q171. What are the Osmotic laxatives or purgatives and how do they work?

Osmotics cause fluids to flow in a special way through the colon, resulting in bowel distention. This class of drugs is useful for people with idiopathic constipation. They include some magnesium and sodium salt and lactulose. Lactulose is a semisynthetic carbohydrate preparation from sucrose and lactose and is not digested or absorbed in the small intestine. It retains water more in the large intestines as it is broken down to more active compounds by the colon bacteria. This has become very popular in recent days. People with diabetes, high BP should be monitored for electrolyte imbalances when they take salts. The commercial preparations of lactulose are Duphalac, Bulky, Agrolac, Fressh, Livo Luk, Safex. Milk of magnesia also falls in osmotic laxatives.

Q172. What are the Stool softeners and how do they work ?

Stool softeners moisten the stool and prevent dehydration. These laxatives are often recommended after childbirth or surgery.These products are suggested for people who should avoid straining in order to pass a bowel movement. The prolonged use of this class of drugs may result in an electrolyte imbalance. This group includes Docusates.

Q173. What are the Lubricant laxatives and how do they work?

Lubricants grease the stool, enabling it to move through the intestine more easily. Mineral oil is the most common example. Commercially available drugs which contain lubricants are Agarol, Cremaffin, laxina, Momplus, Neolax. Liquid paraffin as such can be taken as a lubricant laxative. Lubricants typically stimulate a bowel movement within 8 hours.

> Liver acts as a blood iron buffer and iron storage medium. It stores 60% of excess of iron mainly in form of ferritin and partly as haemosiderin.

Q174. What is the plant Mucus bassorin series?

These chemicals have a very strong swelling capacity in the alkaline environment of small intestine and therefore leads to very strong peristalsis of the intestinal muscles and lead to expulsion of the stool. Two commercially available preparations are Evacuol, Kanormal and they are in tablet form.

Q175. What are the herbal preparations?

Many herbal laxative preparations are now commercially available. Most of them include combinations of naturally occurring herbs. Nityam, Kayam churn, Herbolax, Consticare,

Lexolite, Piles cure, Pilet, Pilovan, Sify, Termilax are some of the available preparations. They use Hartaki,Bael, Senna leaves, Sannoy, Sounth, Pipli,Giloy, Ajwain, Amla, Moti pisth, Saunf, Isobgol,Mullathi, Rose petals, Kala namak, saindhav namak, Phatkari as ingredients in different proportions. Trifala – a preparation of Harkati, Bahera and Amla is also a known herbal preparation for treating constipation.

Q176. What are Enemas and locally acting drugs used in Constipation?

> Liver helps in thermo regulation as it produces large amount of heat.

In Enema – different types of stimulant Chemicals are pushed into the anus and rectum by using tubes made of plastic or rubber. These drugs have astringent, antiseptic or vasoconstrictor effects. In severe constipation enemas can treat the patients successfully. Water enema is also given in many places, in naturopathy centers. Anal suppositories are also used in many cases. In cases of painful anal conditions local creams are also available commercially.

Commercially available enemas are Mesacol Enema, Sulabh enema.

Q177. What can be other treatments of Constipation in special cases?

Treatment for constipation may be directed at a specific cause. For example, the doctor may recommend discontinuing medication or performing surgery to correct an anorectal problem such as rectal prolapse, a condition in which the lower portion of the colon turns inside out.

People with chronic constipation caused by anorectal dysfunction can use biofeedback to retrain the muscles that control bowel movements. Biofeedback involves using a sensor to monitor muscle activity, which is displayed on a computer screen, allowing for an accurate assessment of body functions. A health care professional uses this information to help the patient learn how to retrain these muscles.

Surgical removal of the colon may be an option for people with severe symptoms caused by colonic inertia. However, the benefits of this surgery must be weighed against possible complications, which include abdominal pain and diarrhoea.

Q178. What is the main Dietary management of Constipation?

Management of constipation lies in developing regularity of habit through a bowel training programme and by establishing good healthy habits such as regular meals and elimination timings, adequate fibre and fluid intake and sufficient exercise.

The mainstay of the treatment of constipation is however dietary in nature with a lot of emphasis on dietary fiber and fluid intake. So let us get to know about dietary fiber – the sources and potential benefits.

Dietary fiber is defined as plant polysaccharides resistant to hydrolysis by the digestive enzymes in the human intestinal tract. It includes:

> The small intestine is presented with about 9 L of fluid per day- 2 L from dietary sources and 7 L of gastrointestinal secretions, however, only 1-2 L passes into the colon.

- Structural polysaccharides (insoluble fibre) of the plant cell wall such as cellulose, hemicellulose, non-carbohydrate material, lignin etc.
- Non-structural polysaccharides (soluble fibre) such as pectins, gums and mucilages.

Q. 179. What are the sources of dietary fiber in our diet?

The sources of dietary fiber include whole grain cereals, legumes, whole pulses, leafy vegetables, vegetables like peas, beans, ladies finger, fruits like guava, apple, citrus fruits, nuts, oilseeds like flaxseeds, methi seeds etc.

Q 180. What about the fluid and other nutrient intake during Constipation?

The fluid intake should be at least 2 litres daily. This includes fluids as foods and beverage besides water. The intake of lemon juice, citrus fruit juices, coconut water, vegetable soups, watery dal, lassi and watermelon juice may have an added benefit of adding vital nutrients like potassium which improve the muscle tone.

As for other nutrients i.e. calories, proteins, carbohydrates and fat the requirements would be the same.

The nutritional management should aim at

- Developing regularity of habits of evacuation
- Following a regular and balanced meal pattern
- Consuming a high fibre and adequate fluid diet and
- Increase in physical activity and exercise.

The requirements in constipation is essentially a normal balanced diet with modification in fibre and fluid intake. The intake of fibre should be increased.

Q181. What Yoga will help in Constipation?

These are specific yoga poses for relieving and preventing Irritable Bowel Syndrome (IBS) symptoms, as well as other digestive problems like Constipation.

It is always best (and safest) to learn poses in person from a trained yoga instructor. If you're completely new to yoga try attending local classes first, then supplement your class practices with routines at home. Daily practice will give the best results.

VAJRASANA

Posture

Like Padmasana, this is also the Asana for meditation. One can sit comfortably for a prolonged period in this Asana.

Pre Position

Sitting Position.

Procedure

1.	Fold the left leg in the knee and place the toe on the floor.
2.	Fold the right leg in the knee and place the toe on the floor and join the two toes.
3.	Sit on the pit formed by the parted heels.
4.	Place the palms on the knees.

Position

It is important to keep the spine, the neck and the head, upright in one straight line in this Asana. Keep the sight fixed at the level of the height. Don't have any pressure on the hands. The whole weight of the body be set on the spine. Continue smooth breathing, when the final position is attained.

Releasing

1.	Remove the palms from the knees and bring them to the sides.
2.	Take out the left leg and straighten it.
3.	Take out the right leg and straighten it.
4.	Take the sitting position.

AGNISAR :

Agnisar is the 4th step of pranayama package. Following are the steps for agnisar:

- Sit in Padmasana and keep the hands on the knees in a comfortable position. Close the eyes slightly and concentrate on the mind with normal breathing.
- Exhale slow, deep and stable breathe. Stop the breathe outside, i.e., do Bahirmukh. Stretch both the hands straight and keep them on the knees with slight pressure. Contract and expand the stomach. Try to touch the navel deep inside the stomach.
- Keep the stomach and hands normal before doing poorak i.e., inhale. Now take deep, stable and slow breathe.
- This is one cycle of Agnisar pranayama. In one cycle contract and expand the stomach at least ten times. Increase the number to 30. In the beginning practice it for 5 times and then slowly increase is it up to 15 cycles. During winters you can practice it for 25 cycles. Breathe normally, rest for some time and then do Shavasana.

SUPTA BADDHA KONASANA

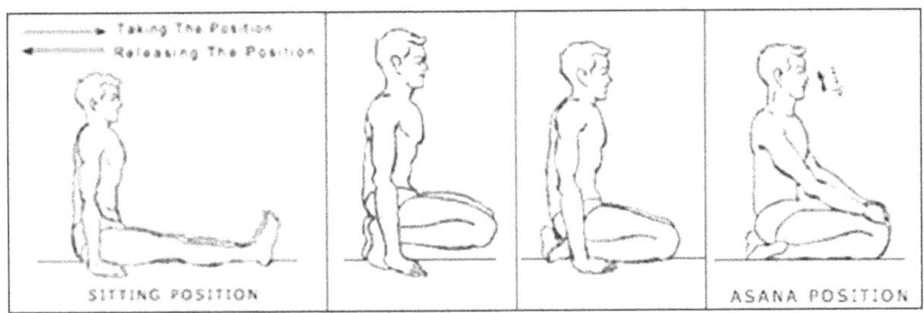

Method

1. Sit in badhha konasana.
2. Slowly lie on the back so that your back & head touches the floor
3. With the help of hands hold ankles & pull them up, so that the heels touches anal region.

4. Put both hand below thighs with palm facing to upwards.
5. Try to touch your knees to the floor.
6. Maintain the pose for 60 secs & breath normally.
7. Exhale & return to original position.

BHUJANGASANA

Bhujangasana makes the spine flexible, removes constipation, and prevents Arthritis. The lungs become strong. Bhujangasana should be practiced along with Shalabhasana and Dhanurasana for deriving maximum benefit. Bowel movement is free and you will not suffer from any major old age problems. You can maintain good shape of the body throughout the life span.

Steps

- Lie down on the floor, belly touching the floor, legs together, toes stretched backwards.

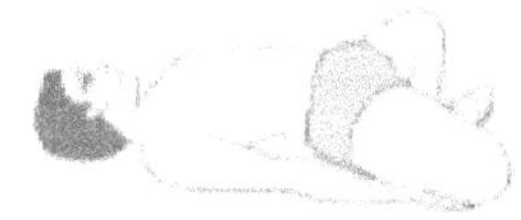

- Keep the palms near the chest and bend the head and the back upwards in a coverage position.
- Bending backwards is more important that lifting the body.
- Inhale and remain in this posture as long as you can hold the breath and then relax.
- Repeat this asana three to six times.

PASCHIMOTTANASANA

(Back spine stretching pose)

Method-

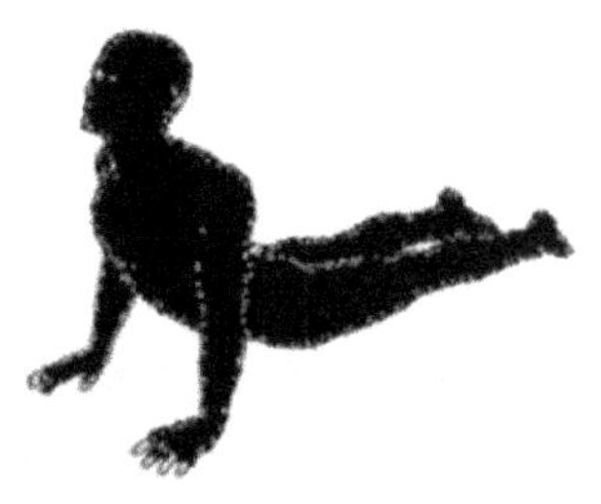

1. Sit in Dandasana.
2. Exhale and lean forward, hold the toes with the help of hands (hold the feet in the middle of the sole.

3. Move more further/forward and downwards from hip to legs.
4. Try to touch your head or nose in between the knees.
5. Do not force yourself to touch your head to knee.
6. You can take folded blanket on knee and touch your head to the blanket.

Durations and Repetitions-

1. Maintain the pose for 20 to 30 secs.
2. Repeat it for 1 to 2 times.

SHASHANKASANA:

This asana strengthens the muscles of the legs and thighs and makes them supple. It tones up the spinal nerves and helps in relieving arthritic pain. It is an excellent asana for digestion. To perform shashankasana following steps can be followed

- Sit with legs folded backwards, heels apart, knees and toes together.
- Adjust your hips between the heels (Vajrasana). Slowly raise your arms over the head.

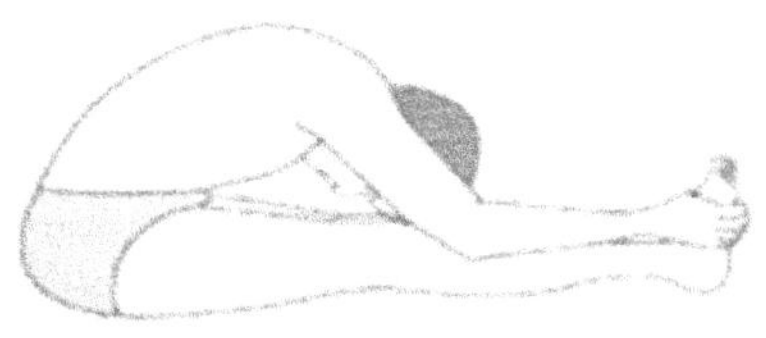

- While exhaling, slowly bend forward and stretch your palms on the floor with abdomen pressing against the thighs.
- Then bring your face downwards and touch the floor with the forehead without raising the buttocks. Inhaling slowly, return to an upright position, reversing the process.

TRIKONASANA

Posture

In this asana the position of the body becomes like a triangle (trikon). And hence, it is called Trikonasana.

Procedure

- Lift the left leg and place it at a maximum distance towards the left

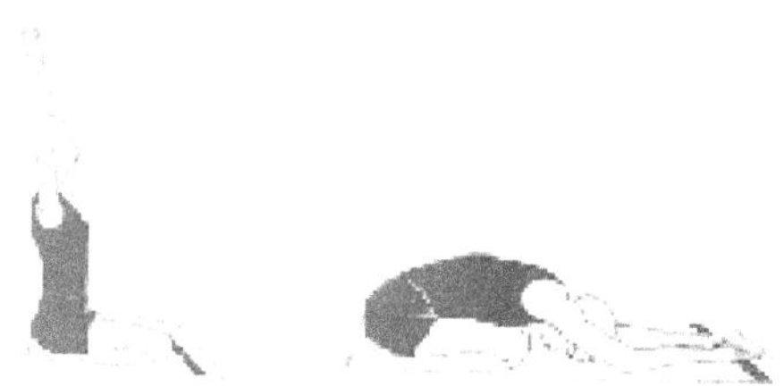

- Turn the toe of the left foot towards the left and inhale.
- Exhale and bend the left leg in the knee and place the left hand palm near the left foot toe.
- Take the right hand forward straight above the right ear and continue smooth breathing.

Position

It is necessary to keep the right hand, mid body and right leg in one straight line in this asana. The neck and the waist should be kept straight. The arms of the right hand should be kept touching the right ear. At this stage, the left leg is kept bent at 90 degree angle, the left arm is kept straight & its palms placed on the floor. In this position the weight of the whole body comes on the left hand. Releasing

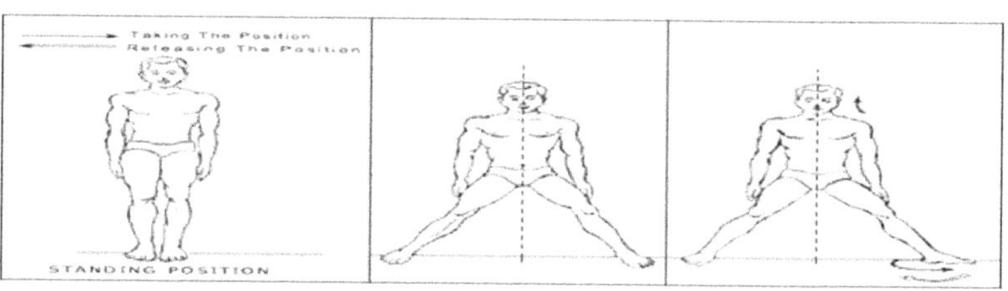

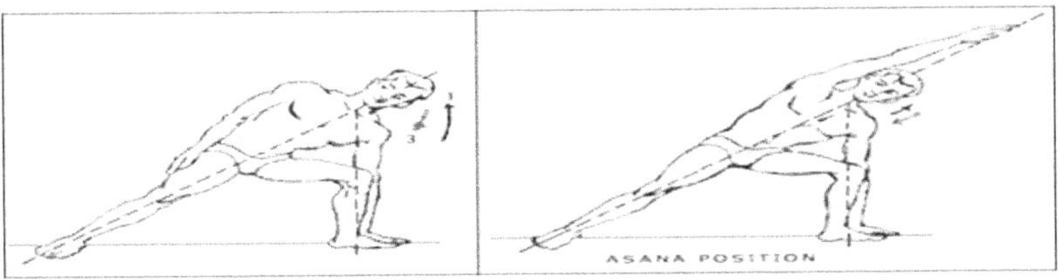

- Exhale and inhailing, bring the right hand to its original place.
- Straighten the left knee and bring the left hand to its original place
- Turn the left leg toe to front.
- Bring the left leg near the right one and take up the standing position.

Duration

It should be kept for one minute on each side.

PAVANMUKTASAN

Method-

1. Lie on back. Exhale and bend both knees. Hold both knees with locked hands.
2. Press thighs gently towards lower abdomen.
3. Raise head up and touch forehead to knees.
4. Maintain the pose upto 30-60 secs and breathe normally.
5. Inhale and return to original pose.

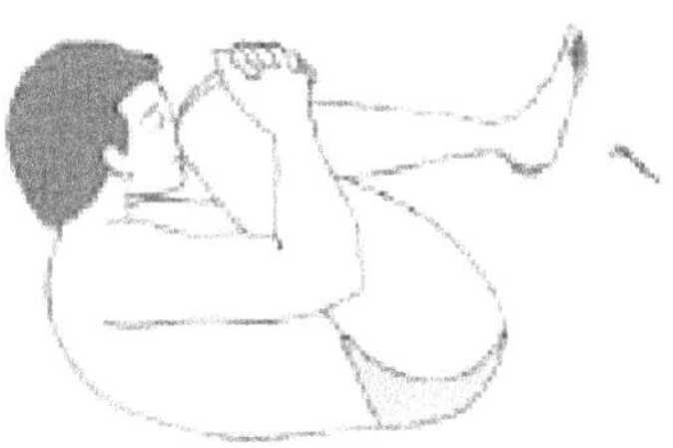

Q182. What is the treatment of Constipation and colitis with Sankh Prakshalan ?

- Sankh Prakshalan is a bowel cleansing method by taking a lot of saline water. It acts as a natural laxative and cleans the bowels. It is similar to the movements of water inside a conch. In this process, luke warm water with some salt is given to drink – few glasses at a time. After every water intake sessions, abdominal exercises are performed to propel this water. After some times, more water is given. Liquid stools start passing after one hour or so. The process is repeated till the stool loses its yellow colour and looks like water. This treatment should only be done under the guidance of Naturopathy experts.

Q183. What are the final tips to remember to prevent and treat Constipation?

- Do not disregard the call of nature. Whenever there is an urge to pass stool, you should not restrict it.
- Establish a gastro-colic reflex by drinking 2 glasses of water in the morning. A full stomach promotes movements of the intestines. So drinking water in the morning after you get up helps to establish a gastro-colic reflux which promotes bowel clearance.
- After drinking water stimulate the intestines by doing free hand abdominal exercises. Try to do forward bending in Vajrasana or Agnisar Kriya which are good abdominal exercises.
- Give time to pass stool. Never be in hurry. Keep your patience. A good bowel clearance always require some times.
- Drink 6-8 glasses of water over and above your thirst. This helps in preventing dry stool.
- Increase intake of high fiber foods (whole grains and

pulses, sprouts, green leafy vegetables and fruits.) High fiber in food helps in forming bulk of stool and making it soft.

- Occasional enema can be taken to soften the stool. This will be required in people with chronic constipation who have very dry stool. However don't make it a habit.
- Daily physical exercise helps in regularizing the bowel movements. Exercise in any form is good. Start with walking and then you can do some specific yogic exercises like Agnisar etc.
- Take 3 teaspoons of Isabgol with a cup of lukewarm water at night. It is safe laxative.
- Some studies has shown that green coloured water can help relieving constipation.
- Junk foods are a leading cause of irregular bowels. Therefore, avoid it as far as possible.
- Gentle heat in abdomen stimulates the bowels.
- Generate pressure in abdomen. It is always better to use Indian toilet.
- A yogic posture is good for digestion. It is only asana which can be done after having food. It is very good for digestion.
- Take one teaspoon of honey mixed in lukewarm water. Squeeze half a lemon in it.
- Hot water with salt acts as a purgative.
- Soak methi seeds in water overnight and chew them along with the some water in the morning.
- A combination of amla, harad and badi harad and bali harad called Trifla to be taken with lukewarm water at night.
- Abdominal massage stimulates the bowel.

Chapter - 9

Diarrhoea or Loose Motion

Q184. What is diarrhoea?

Diarrhoea/Diarrhea is characterized by the evacuation of liquid stools, usually exceeding 300 ml, accompanied by an excessive loss of fluids and electrolytes, especially sodium and potassium. It occurs when there is excessively rapid transit of intestinal contents through the small intestine, decreased enzymatic digestion of foods, decreased absorption of fluids and nutrients or increased secretion of fluids into the GI tract.

An episode of diarrhoea can be acute (recent origin) or chronic (extended duration and repeated episodes) in nature.

Q185. What are the causes of Diarrhoea?

Acute Diarrhoea	Chronic Diarrhoea
Heavy metal poisoing eg. Lead, mercury, arsenic	Malabsorption, lesions of anatomic, mucosal or enzymatic origin
Viral infection (rotavirus)	
Bacterial toxin (salmonella, related to food poisoning), bacterial infection (E. coli; shigella)	Metabolic disease such as diabetic neuropathy, Addison's disease.
Drugs (Neomycin, colichine, antibiotics, antacids, chemotherapy, digoxin, sorbitol)	Carcinoma of small intestine and colon
Psychogenic factors	Cirrhosis of liver
Protozoa infection (giardia, lambia, entamoeba histolytica)	Allergy and food sensitivity

It is evident from the table that acute diarrhea generally occurs in association with infections, poisons and drugs. Chronic diarrhea is due to long-term diseases such as malabsorption syndrome, deficiency of the GI secretions, chronic deficiencies etc.

Q186. What are the types of Chronic Diarrhoea?

Some common forms of chronic diarrhea which you may come across while managing other disease condition include:

> The individual smooth muscle fibers in the gastro intestinal tract are between 200 and 500 micrometers in length and 2 and 10 micrometers in diameter, and they are arranged in bundles of as many as 1000 parallel fibers.

- **Osmotic diarrhea:** This kind of diarrhea is caused by the presence of osmotically active substances in the intestinal tract, which in turn favour the drawing of large volumes of water in the gut eg. Diarrhea associate with lactose intolerance, dumping syndrome (multiple syndrome relate to removal of part of stomach).
- **Secretory diarrhea:** It is result of active secretion of electrolytes and water by the intestine epithelium caused by bacteria and viral infections. These in turn lead to the production of exotoxins and increased intestinal hormone secretion.
- **Limited mucosal contact diarrhea:** It results from situations of inadequate mixing of chime (semi liquid mass of food passing through intestine) and inadequate exposure of chime to intestinal epithelium because of destruction and decreased mucosa due to surgical procedure. This type of diarrhea is usually complicated by steatorrhoea (increased amount of fat in feces).

Q187. What are the consequences of Diarrhoea?

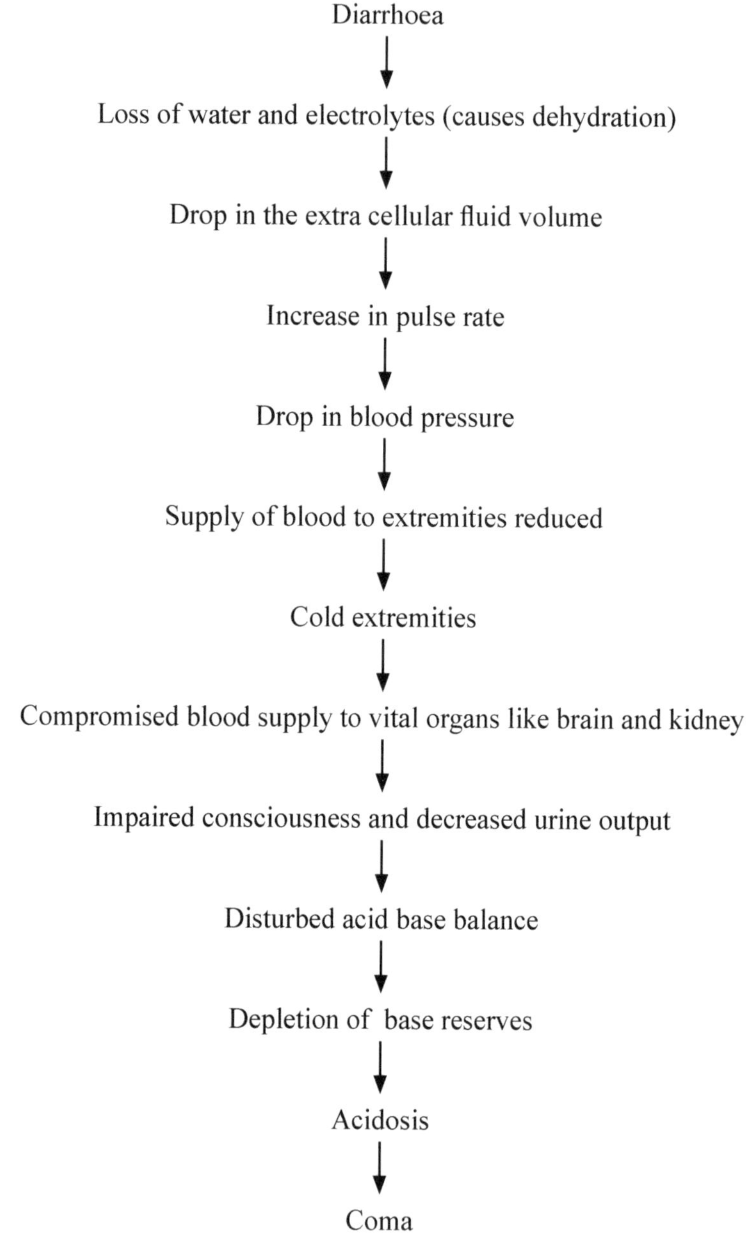

Consequences of Diarrhoea

Q 188. What are the aims in the treatment and management of Diarrhoea?

> The rhythm of contraction of the body of the stomach usually is about 3 per minute of the duodenum about 12 per minute, and of the ileum 8-9 per minute.

Diarrhoea should not be neglected and must received prompt medical care to minimize the frequency of morbidity and mortalities. In light of the complications discussed above, some objectives in the management of the disease should be taken.

Objectives

The major objective in the management of diarrhoea includes:

1. Fluid and electrolyte replacement
2. Removal of cause (especially in case of infection)
3. Nutritional concerns (chronic diarrhoea)

Prompt replacement of fluids and electrolytes is of most significance to prevent morbidities and mortalities associated with dehydration. This is followed by removal of cause through antibiotics, gastric leavage or operative procedure.

For management of diarrhea the first step is to determine the status of dehydration. In mild to moderate cases fluid, electrolyte and acid base should be preserved. Nutritional status should be restored and anti-microbial agents should be given. Associated problems like persistent vomiting, abdominal distension and convulsions should be managed.

Q.189. How to proceed in the real treatment of Diarrhoea?

1. Determining the status of dehydration
2. **Fluid management:** The key to diarrhea management

is the early replacement of fluid lost in the stools through intravenous or oral route. While severe cases need administration of dextrose and electrolyte solution intravenously; mild to moderate cases can be managed at home. The patient can be easily manage by gving fluid at home eg. Coconut water, buttermilk, salted rice kanji, lemon sugar salt beverage or weak tea. This is commonly referred to as the Oral Rehydration Therapy.

- **Oral Rehydration Therapy (ORT):** Homemade/ commercial Oral Rehydration Salts (ORS): refers to providing fluids and/or oral rehydation salt solutions to the patient. An oral rehydration solution can easily be prepared at home by taking a teaspoon of salt 3 tablespoon of sugar with or without lemon juice mixed in a liter of potable water. ORS is also available commercially in small packets.

3. **Emergency treatment and drug management:** Appropriate drugs should be used to treat the cause of diarroea. Severe dehydration is fatal and requires intravenous fluids and hence hospitalization.

Q 190. What are the Nutritional management of Diarrhoea?

Dietary recommendations during diarrhea should take into account the normal recommended dietary intake and various adjustments made to the quality and quantity of the food to be given. The following information will help you understand these concepts.

Energy: During acute phase of diarrhea, the caloric intake can be increased gradually as per the tolerance of the patient. An increment of 200-300 kcal is a

> Under normal resting membrane potential average about 56 milli volts, but multiple factors can change this level.

feasible target. Patient suffering from diarrhea should never be starved as even in acute diarrhea digestive enzymes are functional and almost 60% digestion can take place. Resting the gut can be more damaging as it can bring about structural changes in the gut membrane, which can predispose an individual to associated complication. Calories can be provided through easily digestible carbohydrates. Excess sugar may be avoided to prevent fermentative effect, which may aggravate diarrhea.

Protein: Requirements are only increased in chronic diarrhea because of associated tissues depletion. An additional of 10 gram protein may be recommended above the normal requirements. Milk, a source of good quality protein, is restricted as it is high in residue food or if it is anticipated that diarrhea may have developed due to relative deficiency of lactase in the gastrointestinal tract. Milk in the fermented form like curds is better tolerated, as it is easy to digest and helps in maintaining the gut health. Other cooked and diluted milk products like light porridge; paneer etc can also be tolerated in small amounts.

Fats: Total amount of fat may be restricted as its digestion and absorption is compromised. In order to increase the calorie density of the diet, emulsified fats or those, which are rich in medium chain triglycerides may be added in restricted amounts. Fats like butter, ghee, and cream are easily digested. Fried foods must be avoided. Invinsible form of fat i.e. fat present inherently in the food (egg yolk, whole milk, paneer, curd, flesh food etc.) is tolerated more as compared to visible form of fat.

Carbohydrates: Adequate amount of carbohydrate should be given to the patient. Easily assimilated carbohydrates i.e. principally starches should be preferred. Glucose, sugar, honey, jaggery, potato, yam, rice, sago, semolina, refine flour and pasta can be incorporated to prepare dishes such as khichdi, vegetable/pulse puree, fruit juices, shakes, custard and kanji. The fiber content of the diet should be kept minimum and insoluble fiber should particularly be avoided. A low residue low fiber diet limits the amount of food waste that has to move through the large intestine. These diet may help control diarrhea and abdominal cramping and make eating more enjoyable.

Fiber: Insoluble fibre in the form of skins, seeds should be strictly avoided to minimize the irritation of the GI tract. Soluble fiber in the form of stewed fruits and vegetables like apple juice, stew, guava nectar and pomegranate juice help in binding the stool and favour good environment in the gut. Fruits like papaya and banana have an astringent property and are beneficial.

Vitamins and Minerals: Loss of vitamins is related to the degree of mucosal damage in chronic diarrhea, which in turn impair absorption and synthesis of various essential substances in the body. The vitamins of importance are B complex vitamin especially folic acid, vitamin B12 and vitamin C. Fat soluble vitamin (A, D, E and K) can be lost if fat is not digested and lost in stools. Minerals which are of importance include iron especially if there is an associated bleeding. Sodium and potassium may need to be replaced. Potassium supplementation may favour bowel motility and build up appetite.

Fluids: Intake should be liberal to minimize the risk of dehydration. Preference must be given to diluted drinks as concentrated ones may favour osmotic diarrhoea.

Q191. What are the Low Fibre and Low Residue foods?

Low Fiber Foods

Milk products	Paneer, curd, toned milk
Cereals	Refine cereals, rice, white bread, noodles, maida, suji
Pulses	Dehusked pulses
Vegetables	Potato, bottle gourd, tomato (without skin and seeds), spinach
Fruits	Papaya, banana and fruit juices

Low Residue Foods

Cereals	Rice, refined cereals such as maida, suji, white bread, sweet biscuit, cornflour
Vegetables	Tender, well cooked, pureed low fiber vegetables.
Fruits	Fruit juices or pureed fruits
Meat and its products	Chicken and fish
Pasta	Plain macaroni, noodles, sphagetti etc.
Sweets	White sugar, brown sugar, honey, clear jelly

Q 192. What are the simple tips for prevention of Diarrhoea?

Few simple tips which should be given to the patient:

- Boiling, steaming, baking, pressure cooking should be encouraged.
- Consume small and light meals frequently instead of 3 big meals a day to replenish the lost nutrients.
- Have plenty of fluids like lemon juice, fruit juice, vegetable soups, watery dals, lassi, coconut water etc. to make up for the losses of fluids.
- Have fruits like banana, apple as they are rich in potassium which helps to maintain fluid balance.
- Try to restrict the consumption of milk and dairy

products, as they are difficult to digest.

- Avoid fried foods.
- Avoid raw vegetables like salads.

Golden Rule

- Take food in diarrhea. Don't starve. There are more life lost due to starvation than taking food.
- Take small intervals of meals at 2 hours intervals.
- Give frequent liquids and low residue food.
- Give bland and low fiber diet.

Q 193. What drugs can be used to treat Diarrhoea?

The drugs to treat diarrhoea can be of the following kinds:

a. Anti bacterial drugs
b. Anti Protozoal drugs
c. Combination drugs
d. Probiotics
e. Anti motility drugs
f. Other Anti diarrhoeal drugs

Q194. What are the commercial preparations of such drugs?

a. **Anti bacterials:** Norfloxacin (Norflox), Ciprofloxacin (Ciprobid), Gentamycin, amikacin
b. **Anti Protozoal (anti amoebic, anti gairdia):** Metronidazole, Diloxanide furoate, Tinidazole (Metrogyl, Flagyl, Tini)

c. **Combinations of both** avove are more popular. Some of the examples are Flagyl F, Tini F, Dyrade M, Entamizole, Furoxone, Enteroflox, Norflox TZ, Tiniba N, Electrogyl, Nor metrogyl, Cifran CT, Ciplox TZ. These drugs are very commonly used.

d. **Probiotics:** These drugs have live non harmful germs like lactobacillus (also present in curd, Yogurt). Some preparations are Tanpro, Flora blend, Bifilin etc.

e. **Anti motility drugs:** These are mostly codeine and opium derivatives. Some of the drugs stop the loose motions immediately. Some of the commercially available drugs are Immodium, Lopamide, Lomotil, Lomofen,Lomid.

f. **Other drugs** used for treatment of diarrhoea are Amino salicylic acids(Mesacol), Sulphasalazine (Salazopyrine), Balsalazide (Balacol) . They are used in severe cases or in Ulcerative colitis and Crohn's disease.

Management:
What are to be done by

Patient	Doctors	Practice
Provide ORS to the patient by adding a tsp of salt and 3tsp of sugar in 1 liter of water. One can include emulsified fats like butter, ghee, cream as they are easily digested. Include fluid like soups, juices, curd, coconut water, lemon water in the diet.		✓ Take adequate amount of food do not starve. ✓ Take small intervals of meals. ✓ Restrict total amount of fat. Fried foods must be avoided ✓ Avoid insoluble fiber foods like seeds and skin of fruits. Stew fruits and vegetables can be taken ✓ Take adequate amount of fluid to minimized the risk of dehydration

Chapter - 10

Nausea & Vomiting

Q195. What are Nausea and Vomiting?

The word Nausea comes from a Greek word which means sea sickness. It is an uncomfortable situation which can occur independently or just prior to vomiting. Vomiting is the expulsion of the contents of the stomach and intestine through the mouth. Excess saliva formation, palpitation and urge to defecate often accompany vomiting.

> The gastrointestinal system has a nervous system all its own called the enteric nervous system. It lies entire in the wall of the gut, beginning in the esophagus and extending all the way to the anus. The number of neutrons in this enteric system is about 100 million almost exactly to the number in the entire spinal cord; this demonstrates the importance of the entire system for controlling gastrointestinal functions.

These two are ranked recently as 11th most common reasons to visit an emergency department of hospitals. In healthy persons, the symptoms of nausea and vomiting can be valuable responses as they help to minimize effects of toxins and contaminated food intake. They can be initiated by over eating, pregnancy, motion sickness, after surgery, after cancer treatments, after intake of certain medicines. They can also be caused by diseases like intestinal obstruction, pancreatitis, gastritis, gastroenteritis, peptic ulcer.

Q196. How does vomiting takes place?

Vomiting occurs due to some series of actions in the digestive tract. These are retrograde contraction of the small intestines returning its content to stomach, relaxation of the stomach muscles, opening of the lower sphincter (muscular door) and forceful contraction of the diaphragm and the muscles of the abdomen.

> Cholecystokinin is secreated by "I" cell in the mucosa of the duodenum and jejunum mainly in response to the breakdown product of fat, fatty acids, and monoglycerides in the intestinal contents. It has a potent effect in increasing the contractibility of the gallbladder thus expelling bile into the small intestine, where the bile then plays important role in emulsifying fatty substances, allowing them to digest and absorbed.

There is a vomiting center in the brain which get stimulated when irritants or toxins enter the stomach or distension of the stomach/ intestine takes place. Even drugs and toxins in the blood stream can stimulate the vomiting center. The vestibular organ in the ear, which get over stimulated by repeated abnormal motion (driving in the hills, sailing in the disturbed sea) can also lead to vomiting by stimulation of this brain center. The vomiting center then instructs the nerves to act and complete the vomiting reflex. Vomiting reflex can be stimulated by several receptors like muscarine, dopamine, histamine, serotonin and neurokinin. Many medicines used to treat vomiting block one or more of these recptors.

Q197. How to diagnose the cause of vomiting?

A detailed history of intake of foods just before the vomiting (or nausea) is very important in diagnosis of vomiting. The appearance and the volume of the material coming out can also be very useful. Pain in the abdomen along with vomiting point towards diseases like infection, ulcer etc. Accompanying fever, dehydration, movement of the patient can also give the leads. Finally, medical tests can be done to rule out any disease that may be the cause of vomiting.

Q198. What are the treatments of nausea and vomiting?

The decreased oxygen concentration in the gut wall can increase intestinal blood flow at least 50-100%. Therefore, the increased mucosal and gut wall metabolic rate during gut activity probably lowers the oxygen concentration enough to cause much of the vasodilatation.

The main treatment will be to remove the cause of vomiting. The next is the relief of the problem by appropriate medicines. If the vomiting is prolonged and severe – drugs may have to be given by injection. If there is dehydration – fluids can be given by drip. If there is a history of motion sickness – the motions may be avoided or prior medicines to stop the motion sickness can be given.

Q199. What are the drugs used to treat vomiting?

The drugs are Metoclopramides, Phenothiazines, Butyrophenones, Benzamides, Anti cholinergic drugs, serotonin receptor antagonists and antihistaminics. The commercial preparations of Metoclopramides are Emenil, Perinorm, Reglan, Maxeron, Nausifar. Metoclopramides have anti dopamine action and inhibit vomiting by acting through the brain center.

Chapter - 11

Inflamatory Bowel Disease

Q200. What is Inflamatory Bowel Disease and what are the causes, symptoms and complications of IBD?

The term Inflammatory Bowel Disease (IBD) covers a group of disorders in which the intestines become inflamed (red and swollen), probably as a result of an immune reaction of the body against its own intestinal tissue. The three major type of IBD are:

1. Ulcerative colitis
2. Crohn's disease
3. Short bowel syndrome

When the inflammation is in rectum with extension into the colon without affecting the right colon or small intestine, the disease is called ulcerative colitis. When inflammatory process involves one or more lengthy segments of the small or large intestine with inflammation from the mucosa to serosa, the disease is called Crohn's disease.

The Causes of IBD:

Researchers do not yet know what causes

All the jaws working together can close the teeth with a force as great as 55 pounds on the incisors and 200 pounds on the molars.

inflammatory bowel disease. Therefore, IBD is called an idiopathic disease (disease with an unknown cause).An unknown factor/agent (or a combination of factors) triggers the body's immune system to produce an inflammatory reaction in the intestinal tract that continues without control. As a result of the inflammatory reaction, the intestinal wall is damaged leading to bloody diarrhoea and abdominal pain.

Genetic, infectious, immunologic, and psychological factors have all been implicated in influencing the development of IBD.

Most of the muscles of chewing are innervated by the motor branch of the fifth cranial nerve, and the chewing process is controlled by nuclei in the brain stem.

There is a genetic predisposition (or perhaps susceptibility) to the development of IBD. However, the triggering factor for activation of the body's immune system has yet to be identified. Factors that can turn on the body's immune system include an infectious agent (as yet unidentified), an immune response to an antigen (eg, protein from cow milk), or an autoimmune process. As the intestines are always exposed to things that can cause immune reactions, more recent thinking is that there is a failure of the body to turn off normal immune responses.

Food swallowed by a person who is in the upright position is usually transmitted to the lower end of the esophagus even more rapidly than the peristaltic wave itself, in about 5-8 seconds, because of the additional effect of gravity pulling the food downward.

The Symptoms of IBD:

Because inflammatory bowel disease is a chronic disease (lasting a long-time), you will go through periods in which the disease flares up and causes symptoms. These periods are followed by remission, in which symptoms disappear or decrease and good health returns.

Symptoms may range from mild to severe and generally

depend upon the part of the intestinal tract involved. They include the following:

- Abdominal cramps and pain
- Bloody diarrhea
- Severe urgency to have a bowel movement
- Fever
- Loss of appetite
- Weight loss
- Anemia (due to blood loss)
- Malnutrition

The Complications of IBD:

Pepsin the important peptic enzyme of the stomach is most active at a pH of 2.0-3.0 and is inactive at a pH about 5. Consequently, for this enzyme to cause any digestive action on protein, the stomach juice must be acidic.

Intestinal complications of inflammatory bowel disease include the following:

- Profuse bleeding from the ulcers
- Perforation (rupture) of the bowel
- Strictures and obstruction: In persons with Crohn's disease, strictures often are inflammatory and frequently resolve with medical treatment. Fixed or fibrotic (scarring) strictures may require endoscopic or surgical intervention to relieve the obstruction. In ulcerative colitis, colonic strictures should be presumed to be malignant (cancerous).
- Fistulae (abnormal passage) and perianal disease: These are more common in persons with Crohn's disease. They may not respond to vigorous medical treatment. Surgical intervention often is required, and there is a high risk of recurrence.
- Toxic megacolon (acute non obstructive dilation of

the colon): This is a life-threatening complication of ulcerative colitis and requires urgent surgical intervention. It is fortunately relatively rare.

- Malignancy: The risk of colon cancer in ulcerative colitis begins to rise significantly above that of the general population after approximately 8-10 years of diagnosis. The risk of cancer in Crohn's disease may equal that of ulcerative colitis if the entire colon is involved. The risk of small intestine malignancy is increased in Crohn's disease.

> The total quantity of fluid that must be absorbed each day by the intestines is equal to the ingested fluid (about 1.5 lt) plus that secreted in the various gastrointestinal secretion (about 7 lt). This comes to about 8-9 liters. All but about 1.5 liters is absorbed in the small intestine, leaving only the 1.5 liter to pass through the ileocecal valve into the colon each day.

Extra intestinal complications:

- Extra intestinal involvement of IBD refers to complications involving organs other than the intestines. These affect only a small percentage of people with IBD.
- Persons with IBD may have arthritis, skin conditions, inflammation of the eye, liver and kidney disorders, and bone loss. Of all the extra intestinal complications, arthritis is the most common. Joint, eye, and skin complications often occur together.

Q201. What may be the treatment of IBD?

Self-Care at Home:

It is important to eat a healthy diet. Depending on your symptoms a decrease in the amount of fiber or dairy products in your diet is suitable.

Diet has little or no influence on the inflammatory activity in ulcerative colitis. However, diet may influence symptoms. For this reason, people with inflammatory bowel disease often are placed on a variety of diet interventions, especially low-residue diets. Evidence does not support a low-residue diet as beneficial in treating the inflammation of ulcerative colitis, though it might decrease the frequency of bowel movements.

Absorption from the small intestine each day consist of several hundred grams of carbohydrates, 100 or more gram of fat. 50-100 gram of proteins, 50-100 gram of ions, and 7-8 liters of water. The absorptive capacity of the small intestine is far greater than this: as much as several kilos of carbohydrates/ day, 500g of fat/ day, 500-700 g protein/day and 20 or more liters of water/day.

Unlike ulcerative colitis, diet can influence inflammatory activity in Crohn's disease. Nothing by mouth (NPO status) can hasten reduction of inflammation, as might the use of a liquid diet or a predigested formula.

Less than 0.5 % of the intestinal sodium is lost in the feces each day because of its rapid absorption through the intestinal mucosa. Sodium also plays an important role in helping to absorb sugars and amino acids.

When the patient becomes extremely upset the symptoms may get worse. Therefore, it is important that the patients learn to manage the stresses in life.

About 1500 mililiters of chime normally pass through the ileocecal valve into the large intestine each day. Most of the water and electrolytes in the chyme are absorbed in the colon, usually leaving less than 100 mililiters of fluid to be excreted in the feces.

Medication:

Medications used to treat the symptoms of Crohn's disease include 5-aminosalicylic acid (5-ASA) formulations, prednisone, immunomodulators such as azathioprine, mercaptopurine, methotrexate, infliximab, adalimumab, certolizumab and natalizumab. Hydrocortisone should be used in severe attacks of Crohn's disease.

❑

Health Books by Dr. Bimal Chhajer

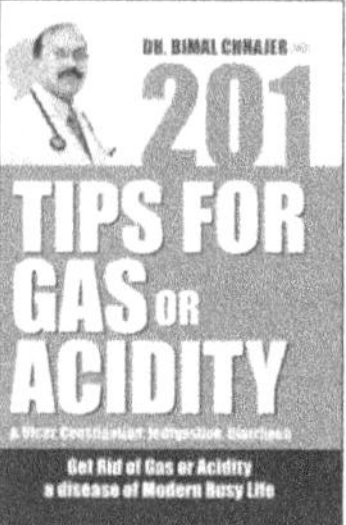

201 Tips for Gas Acidity

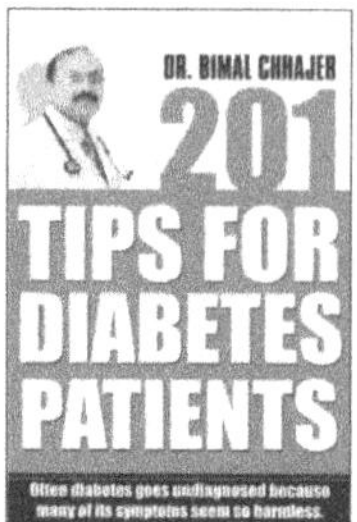

201 Tips for Diabetes Patients

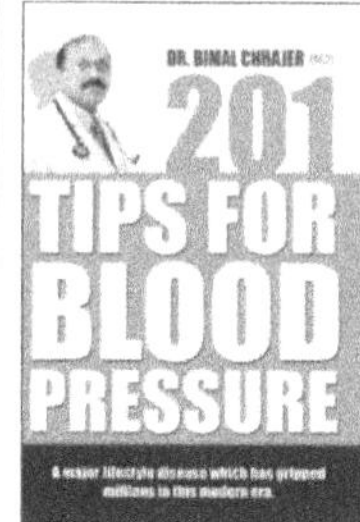

201 Tips For Blood Pressure

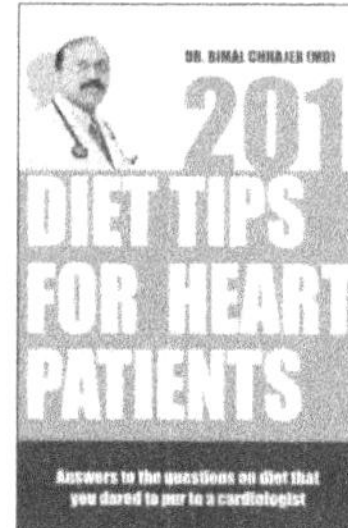

201 Diet Tips for Heart Patients

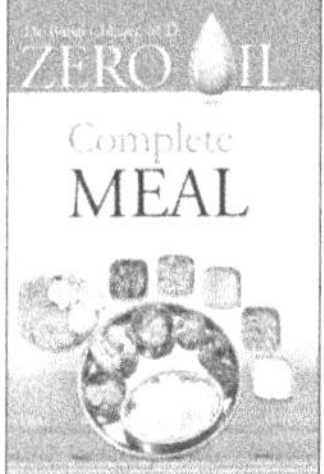

Zero Oil Complete Meal

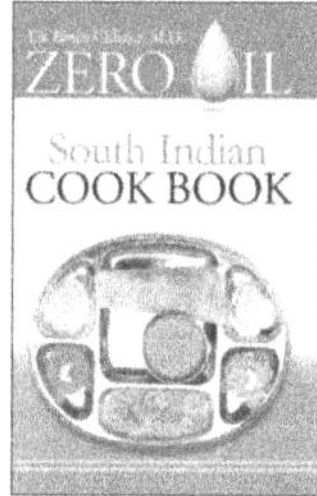

Zero Oil South Indian Cook Book

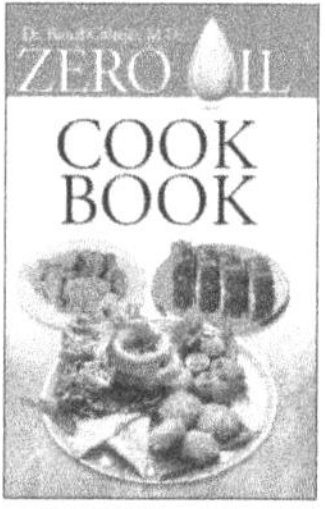

Zero Oil Cook Book

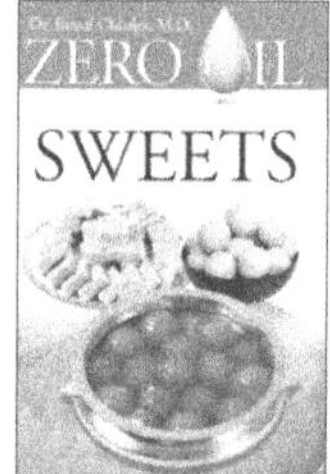

Zero Oil Sweets

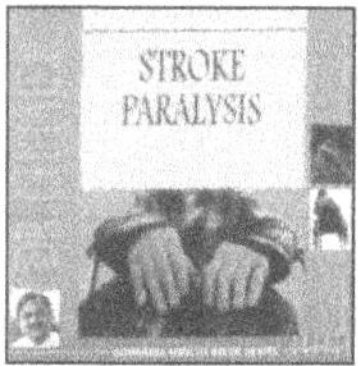

Stroke Paralysis

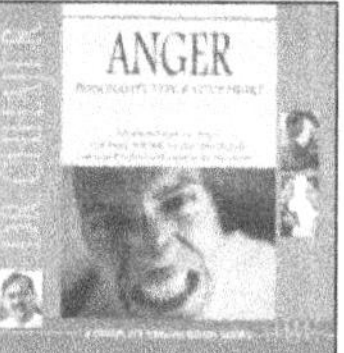

Anger

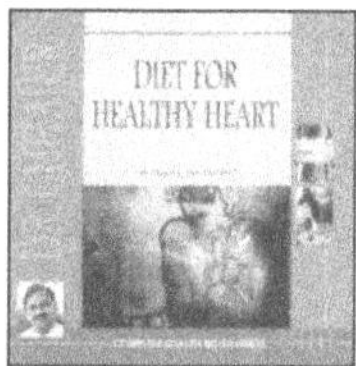

Diet for Healthy Heart

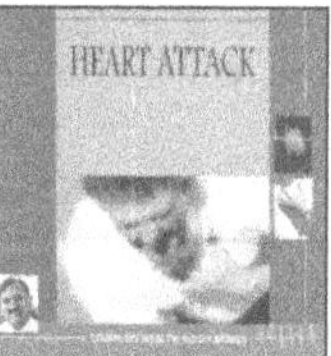

Heart Attack

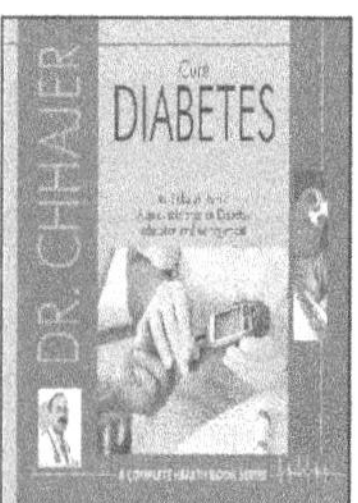

Diabetes

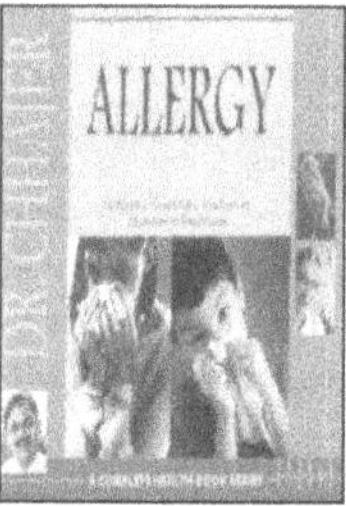

Allergy

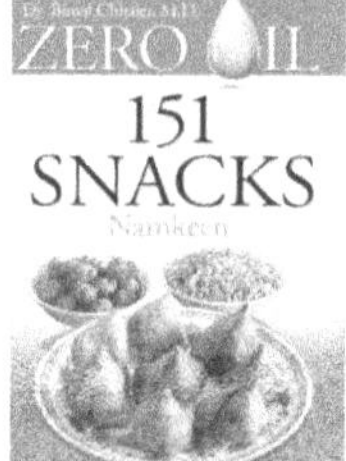

Zero Oil 151 Snacks

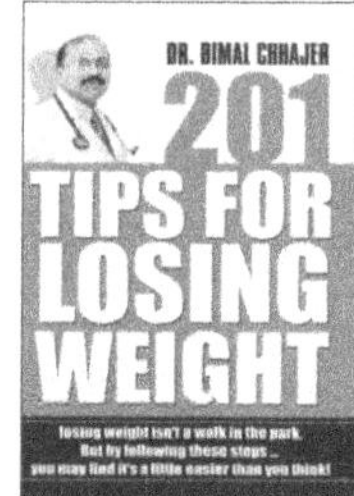

201 Tips For Loosing Weight

www.ingramcontent.com/pod-product-compliance
Ingram Content Group UK Ltd.
Pitfield, Milton Keynes, MK11 3LW, UK
UKHW021659190726
13853UKWH00001B/358

9 789350 833094